Eye Disease in the Tropics

Eye Disease in the Tropics

A PRACTICAL TEXTBOOK FOR DEVELOPING COUNTRIES

F.C. Rodger
MD, ChM, FRCS(G), DOMS

Senior Consultant Ophthalmic Surgeon,
Princess Margaret Hospital, Swindon.

Member, WHO Expert Advisory Panel
on Parasitic Diseases (Filarial Infections).

Formerly Professor of Ophthalmology,
Aligarh University, India, and Director, British West African Blind Surveys.

Foreword by

A.W. Woodruff
CMG, MD, PhD, FRCP, FRCPE, DTM&H

Wellcome Professor of Clinical & Tropical Medicine,
London School of Hygiene & Tropical Medicine.

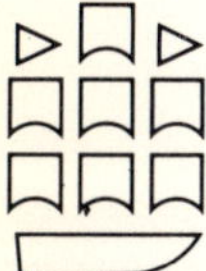

CHURCHILL LIVINGSTONE
EDINBURGH LONDON MELBOURNE AND NEW YORK 1981

CHURCHILL LIVINGSTONE
Medical Division of Longman Group Limited

Distributed in the United States of America by Churchill
Livingstone Inc., 19 West 44th Street, New York, N.Y. 10036,
and by associated companies, branches and representatives
throughout the world.

© Longman Group Limited 1981

First published 1981

ISBN 0 443 02020 5

British Library Cataloguing in Publication Data
Rodger, Frederick Carson
    Eye disease in the tropics.
    1. Tropics – Diseases and hygiene
    2. Eye – Diseases and defects
    I. Title
    617'.7'091'3   RE46   80-49725

Printed in Singapore by Kyodo Shing Loong Printing Industries Pte Ltd

Foreword

Blindness is one of the great medical problems in the world today. Latest estimates indicate that there are 28 000 000 people who cannot count fingers at a distance of 3 metres. The problem is greatest in tropical regions for there, onchocerciasis, leprosy, malnutrition causing xerophthalmia and trachoma are major causes of blindness which are either not present in temperate regions or are uncommon there. There are also common hereditary diseases such as sickle cell anaemia in which ophthalmic complications are common. Eye disease is therefore something with which all practitioners in the tropics will come in contact, either as an expression of more general disease or as a condition of which the presenting manifestation is ophthalmic. Yet there are many gaps in the knowledge of ophthalmology possessed by most practitioners in tropical regions. The undergraduate medical curriculum is so crowded that ophthalmology like other specialities is given but a small allocation of time. Even those who qualify in the tropics find large gaps in their knowledge and those who go from temperate regions to practice medicine in the tropics almost invariably find that for a year or two there are many fields in which they have to grope.

There are numerous books on ophthalmology but few on the special tropical manifestations of the subject and fewer still in which the common ophthalmic diseases in the tropics are given prominence together with the means of managing them, whereas the setting up of a diagnostic laboratory for ophthalmology in the tropics is something which even experienced ophthalmologists in temperate regions would find difficult. Mr F.C. Rodger has great experience in all these fields and his book is designed to give practical help to all practitioners in the tropics or proceeding to the tropics, not only ophthalmic specialists but also all medical officers, physicians or surgeons working there.

There is a great need for a book of this kind and Mr Rodger is very well qualified to write it. During the past 30 years he has made many expeditions to the tropics and has spent long periods there investigating ophthalmic disease; his innumerable very important contributions to the literature on the subject cover a wide range of tropical ophthalmology. In all his work the practical approach is emphasised. In the world today there are none more qualified and few as qualified as he is to write a book of this kind. In bringing this work to completion he has performed a great service, not only to medicine and the medical community but to humanity. The book deserves success and will surely be a valued addition to all libraries and connections of those working in the tropics.

London, 1981　　　　　　　　　　　　A.W. Woodruff

Preface

The subject of ophthalmology has for many years been recognised as a vital one in tropical countries, so much so that in most it is a compulsory subject in the final year medical examinations. In recent years, with the compression of lines of communication, and man's increasing preparedness to visit and help his neighbour, tropical eye diseases as a subject has come very much to the fore in temperate climates as well.

The object of this book is to give, as shortly but as comprehensively as possible, accounts of those eye diseases of greatest importance and most common occurrence. In addition, practical information is listed as to what to expect on arriving in a strange land, what instruments and medicines to take and how to commission, if it is possible, a small diagnostic laboratory.

The book is intended for medical men who work with few facilities in areas often remote, yet with dense populations. It should also be of help to medical students and to those who teach nurses and paramedicals. Some of the doctors—reared in, or with experience of, the tropics—may have no ophthalmic training; others may be qualified ophthalmologists but newcomers to the third world. In consequence, overlapping of information, necessary to one and known by the other, has on occasion been unavoidable. The aim has always been to supply a textbook covering most eventualities for those who only too often work alone.

As the development of so many underdeveloped countries progresses, so the quality of clinical medicine (and ophthalmology) in these countries must progress too. Lord Macaulay has said 'Knowledge advances by steps; and not by leaps!' It is hoped this book fulfils that predication.

Shipton Moyne, F.C.R.
Gloucestershire, 1981

Acknowledgements

The author has found the advice of the following colleagues of inestimable value in the expression of opinions or formulation of the text; in particular he is grateful to Dr Bill Crewe and Mr J.E. Friend, whose technical laboratory procedures (for the Liverpool School of Tropical Medicine) make up the bulk of Chapter 7. The author's gratitude is no less in the case of help received from:

Dr J.E. Agar, Princess Margaret Hospital, Swindon.
Dr S.G. Browne, Leprosy Study Centre, London.
Dr A. Buck, Princess Margaret Hospital, Swindon.
Dr H.C. Drysdale, Princess Margaret Hospital, Swindon.
Dr J.A. Waddell, Princess Margaret Hospital, Swindon.
Dr Wendell Wilson, Louisiana State University Medical Center.

Above all, I am grateful to my secretary, Mrs Margaret Stephens, for her efficiency, speed, interest and understanding in preparing the manuscript. Thanks are also due to Miss H.L. Spurrier of Princess Margaret Hospital Library for checking the references.

The author gratefully acknowledges permission to reproduce certain illustrations, as follows:

Scientific Exploration Society for the Frontispiece.
Professor Y. BenSira, Beilinson Hospital, Tel Aviv (Plate 7).
Dr D.P. Choyce, Hospital for Tropical Diseases, London (Plates 2, 16, 20, 21, 27, 28, 34, 48).
Dr W. Crewe, School of Tropical Medicine, Liverpool (Plates 43, 44, 47).
Dr K.D. Crow, Princess Margaret Hospital, Swindon (Plate 53).
Dr D.W. Ellis-Jones, Memorial Hospital, Crewe, and British Journal of Ophthalmology (Plate 52).
Professor P.E.C. Manson-Bahr, Ministry of Overseas Development, London (Plate 40).
Professor E. Neumann, Rothschild University Hospital, Haifa (Plate 33).
Mr K.S. Sehmi, Moorfields Eye Hospital, London (Plate 41).
Dr J.D. Strong, Princess Margaret Hospital, Swindon (Plates 29, 35, 36, 37).
Dr D.A. Warrell, John Radcliffe Hospital, Oxford (Plates 14 and 54).
Dr K.S. Zinn and Dr S.L. Guillory, Mount Sinai Hospital, New York (Plate 51).
Author and Experimental Eye Research (Plate 18).
Author and Hutchinson, London (Plate 8).
Author and Lewis, London (Plates 12 and 30).
World Health Organisation (Plate 9).
Author and Acta Ophthalmologica (Plate 18).
Author and American Journal of Ophthalmology (Plates 19 and 22).
Author and British Journal of Ophthalmology (Plates 6 and 39).
Author and Pergamon Press, Oxford (Plates 4, 23 and 24).

The rest of the photographs and the drawings are the work of the author, who is grateful to Mr St John A.F. Fallows, the Director, and staff of the Department of Photography, Princess Margaret Hospital, Swindon, for preparing them for publication.

*This book is dedicated to my wife, Jess,
who has travelled many rough roads with me.*

Contents

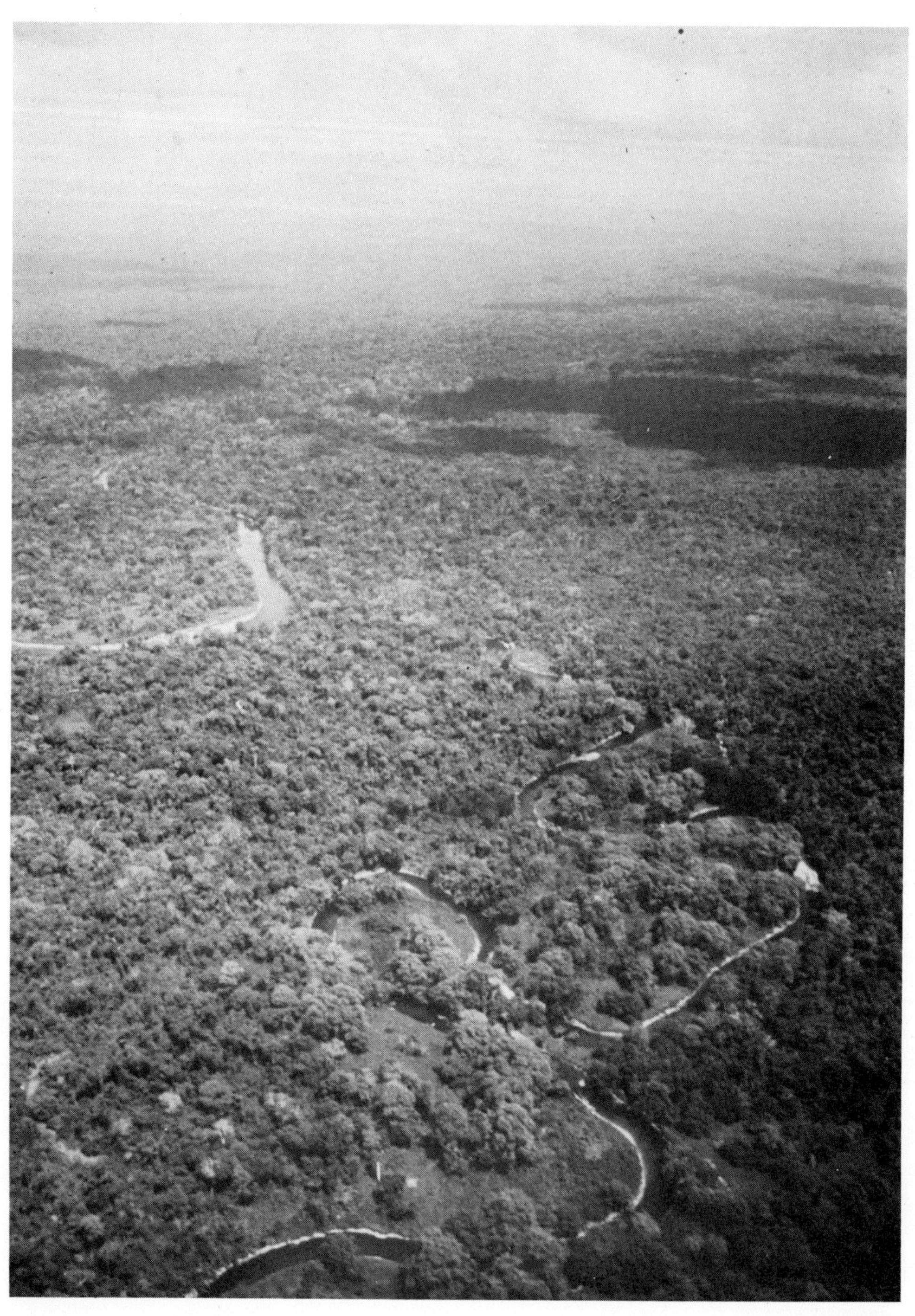

Frontispiece In the Zaire forest can be found most ocular diseases. Trachoma, unexpectedly, is rare or absent

1

Preparatory planning

The international classification of blindness, the technique of measuring vision and information needed to collect data on prevalence rates of blindness acceptable under international standards are supplied in this chapter.

Details of the simplest basic ophthalmic equipment are listed and, for the benefit of non-ophthalmologists, how best to use them.

Certain eyedrops and ointments, drugs and their usages are given as a guide to what may be required and ordered beforehand. The least costly are selected wherever possible, but where only the expensive are likely to be useful, these also are listed.

VISUAL STANDARDS

Measurement of visual acuity

Until standards of blindness are universal there can be no direct comparison between the incidence or prevalence rates of blindness between different countries. If the visual acuity is recorded for each eye separately, more realistic data will be obtained of the ocular damage done than if binocular acuity alone were to be considered in eye disease.

When measuring vision in illiterates the usual test is to give the patient a separate large letter capital 'E' (corresponding in size with 6/60 on the Snellen chart), asking him to move it into positions which correspond to those indicated by the letter which the examiner points to on the chart. An alternative is to ask the patient to point in the direction to which the letter points. As it is often possible to guess where the three legs of a capital 'E' are directed, without being certain whether it is pointing up or down, or right or left, use of the Landolt 'ring' or capital 'C' is a more

acceptable test target to the visual physiologist; here the patient indicates with his finger, or with a model letter, in which direction the gap in the ring occurs, and to do so the gap must be seen; he simply cannot guess.

The test is best carried out in daylight with the patient's back to the sun so that he is not dazzled, the eyes being tested singly, and then both together. The investigator holds the Snellen chart of Landolt 'Cs' 6 metres away, each intervening metre being marked on the ground. The subject is asked to indicate with his fingers where the gap is. If the top letter (marked 60 beneath; sometimes marked above) is seen, but no others, then visual acuity is recorded as 6/60. If the top letter at 6 m is not seen, then a large letter which corresponds in size to 6/60 is taken by the examiner, who moves it into different positions at each of the intervening metre stages. In practice he can cut the corners a bit by carrying out this procedure at 3m and 1m only; this will permit him to classify any visual impairment in accordance with WHO recommendations.

When the patient is not able to see the letter at 1 m (1/60), then he is taken into a dark room and light is projected into each eye in turn. If the light is seen, then the patient has to indicate from which quadrant of the visual field it comes. On completing this test then the perception of light is recorded as being either 'well projected' or 'not well projected'.

Classification of blindness

In the publication 'International Classification of Diseases (1979)', the following classification of blindness is given (Table 1.1). It is based on six categories of visual loss and it can be seen by reference to the previous section that all the information required can be gained by the technique recommended there. This classification resulted from a WHO Report (Bietti et al, 1972) stressing the need to prevent blindness and standardise procedures.

seen than with white light.

Green light (439 to 548 nm) has been used widely for a long time because of its clarification of surface features. Oedema and reflexes from the surface of the

Table 1.1 WHO classification of blindness

Category	Binocular visual acuity	Professional independence	Social independence
1	6/18–6/60	Yes	Yes
2	6/60–3/60 (i.e. counts fingers at 3m, CF at 3m)	No	Yes
3	3/60–1/60 (CF at 3m–CF at 1m)	No	Yes
4	CF at 1m–PL	No	No
5	No PL	No	No
6	Undetermined or unspecified	—	—

To clarify, in Category 1 the patient sees $\frac{6}{18}$ or less up to $\frac{6}{60}$ inclusive, etc.

These categories make it possible to provide prevalence rates of seriously impaired vision (1 and 2) as well as of blindness (3, 4 and 5) for single eyes, or for both eyes taken together.

BASIC EQUIPMENT

Three instruments are vital if eye diseases are to be correctly diagnosed and treated: an ophthalmoscope, a slit lamp (optical biomicroscope) and a tonometer. Others are less vital but helpful.

Ophthalmoscope

Most ophthalmoscopes have three (increasingly wide) apertures for white light, but it has been found extremely useful to have an ophthalmoscope with three apertures of the same (medium) size, one for white light without a filter, one with a green filter and one with a yellow filter.

A yellow filter (588 to 589 nanometers)* allows the observer to see through incipient cataracts and diseased vitreous much better than with white light. The retinal nerve fibres are clearer and, because the retinal pigment is less well seen, details below the surface of the retina, and even within the choroid are better seen. More deeply placed reflexes, as from exudates, are quite well seen, but surface reflexes and scars are not seen; macular details are often better

retina, persistent myelin, gliosis, the shape and form of the optic discs and the retinal blood vessels and haemorrhages are all better delineated with red-free light than with anything else. With these two filter additions to white light (yellow and green) available, the usefulness of the direct ophthalmoscope is greatly increased.

Red light (686 to 705 nm) shows up deep pigment more clearly and this can reveal changes below the macula or around the macula, which are not visible in any other way; this at times is helpful. However, most ophthalmoscopes have only three apertures, and the selection of white, yellow and green is a better selection than red, yellow and green.

Slit lamp

Slit lamps are expensive and bulky, but the hand model made by the KOWA Company of Japan is ideal, especially as it can be readily converted to work off a 12-volt car battery, and is light. It can be used as easily as a hand loupe and torch, and has the added advantage over more conventional models of being suitable for examining the eyes of infants, those who are unable to sit up, and the deformed. If the techniques of gonioscopy and usage of the triple mirror are mastered, both can be carried out quite easily with the KOWA model. A table hanging-stand is available as an accessory. The slit lamp contains a cobalt blue filter. The KOWA slit lamp gives magnifications of × 10 and × 20. In one eyepiece there is a useful graduated glass, each division on the scale

*1 nanometer (nm) = 10 Ångstrom units (Å).

representing 0.05 mm. This is ideal for measuring the diameters of the various pathological lesions which may be seen.

Techniques of biomicroscopy

The use of a focused beam is the basis of all methods used in biomicroscopy except for the first named below.

Direct diffuse illumination. The entire front face of the cornea, iris or lens, is illuminated by bringing a broad beam in at a slight angle, and passing it across the surface under observation. This stereoscopic view is a vast improvement on what one can see with a torch and loupe.

Sclerotic scatter. A fairly narrow beam is focused on the limbus. If the cornea is normal, the light, scattered (that is dispersed) by the non-translucent sclera, will pass sideways through the corneal stroma unimpeded, except for a faint haze at the periphery (scleral spur and/or arcus). Any disturbance of the normal corneal transparency (e.g. a faint scar or blood vessel) is immediately made visible where the light is interrupted. The brightest illumination is required.

Direct focal illumination. If the use of a focused beam is the basis of biomicroscopy, no method is more effective than that of direct focal illumination, where the focal point of the beam is made to coincide with the focus of the microscope. Whereas the cornea seems transparent to direct diffuse illumination, the focused beam reveals this is not quite true; no ocular tissue in fact is completely transparent. Each has a complex cellular structure, which leads to some internal dispersion of light, a feature called 'relucency'. The more dense the optical structure is, the greater is its relucency. Relucency is a measure of the heterogeneity of a medium. There is no relucency in quality glass. Relucency is the opposite of translucency. When a beam is focused on a relatively non-transparent structure, like the sclera, most of the light is reflected, dispersed or absorbed. Relucency is total. If the beam passes through a relatively transparent structure like the cornea, because the inherent relucency is only slight, an opalescent block of light is visible in which abnormalities will be grey or white, as they are more dense. If the abnormalities are fluid, being less dense, the changes are darker than the normal relucent cornea.

Because the beam is passed through the cornea obliquely at an angle, the resulting shape is a rectangular block, the outer and inner surfaces being curved by reason of the convexity of the cornea. The width of this optical block of light (geometrically called a parallelepiped prism) can be varied until the block is either so wide that it gives rise to diffuse illumination, or so thin that it is better called an optical section (Figs 1.1 and 1.2).

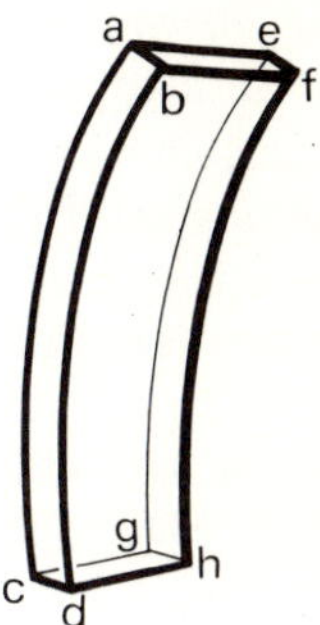

Fig. 1.1 Optical 'parallelepiped', the corneal thickness seen with the slit lamp. The anterior face is marked a b c d, the posterior e f g h

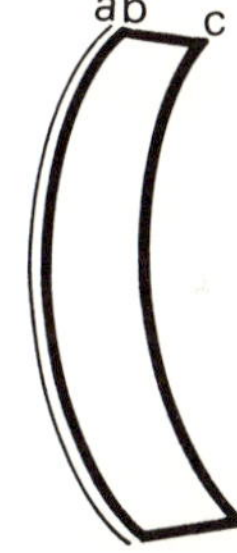

Fig. 1.2 When the slit lamp beam is narrowed, the cornea is seen as an optical 'section' with three layers: a, is the tear film, only seen when fluorescein bathes the cornea; b, is the anterior face of the stroma; c, the posterior face. Normally the area between a and b is optically empty

Between the posterial corneal surface and the anterior lens surface lies the aqueous humor in the anterior chamber, which—provided it is healthy—should be optically empty, and having a low optical density will appear dark.

The lens structure can be similarly scrutinised and is seen to be formed of different layers, as is the cornea, although the different lenticular layers are not revealed instantaneously, but gradually as the focus of the optical beam is advanced ever more deeply. The various layers of the lens, having different refractive indices, deviate the direct path of the beam; at these surfaces the beam is also partly reflected. These 'polished' surfaces are known as the *zones or lines of discontinuity*. The major ones are those between the lens capsule and its cortex, and the cortex and the nucleus. Similar reflecting zones, or lines, exist in the cornea at its anterior and posterior stromal surfaces.

Beyond the lens the vitreous fibrillae with deep focusing are seen with difficulty, but well enough to observe floating cells and changes in the fluidity or the density of the vitreous gel if they occur. If the patient is asked to move his eye up, down, sideways and straight, healthy vitreous should cease moving in 1 minute.

By reducing the height and width of the optical beam, the optical block can be made into a thin optical section, then a shorter section, and finally a small round pencil of rays. If the aqueous is proteinous, or inflammatory cells are present, the small pencil of rays will reveal them.

Collation of the appearances seen with different widths, in what is a saggittal view of the anterior structures of the eye, is what provides the highly detailed information the slit lamp affords by direct focal illumination.

Retro-illumination. This simple method describes the view obtained when the beam is focused obliquely on the non-transparent iris or an opaque lens. A great deal of the beam in such circumstances is reflected back through the cornea. If the observer looks to one side of the beam, he will see the cornea illuminated in this way from behind. The colour will no longer be that of white light, as it will reflect to some degree the colour of the reflecting surface. In the Negro eye this is particularly noticeable.

This is a good method to use routinely when looking for corneal epithelial changes (oedema, vacuoles or posterior precipitates on the cornea, or fine scars at all levels).

Specular reflection. Specular reflection is defined as reflection from a plane where regular reflection occurs as from a mirrored surface. If the eye is aligned with the angle of reflection, it is dazzled; not unexpectedly such reflection occurs at all the zones or lines of discontinuity described above whether from the cornea or from the lens. Irregularities on these different surfaces are discernible because they reflect light irregularly from a surface otherwise reflecting perfectly. This is the main function of the technique. Pathological features involving the zones of discontinuity will then be made manifest and any pathological change in front of the zone of specular reflection, being obstructive, helps in their localisation. Clearly, the fewer the irregularities, that is the more perfect the reflecting surface, the harder it is to be sure exactly where specular reflection is occurring. It reveals changes in the corneal epithelium much better than the techniques of retro-illumination. Repeated re-focusing on each surface is required.

Mini-dark adaptometer

The Rodger mini-dark adaptometer (RDA) has now been tested in Panama, Papua New Guinea and Sulawesi, and found suitable for subjects 8 years of age and upwards. The number of patients to be tested depends on the number of head masks, which have two types of foam lining, one for adults and a second (thicker) for children, that are available. These masks are not expensive. They are fitted over the face and then left in place with the shutter open over the selected eye, the other shutter being closed.

The quality of visual acuity must be known for each eye; vision of 6/18 or better qualifies. Only one eye need be tested. The subjects are each shown, with the least dense filters in position, the target circle with the arrow in the centre, and asked to indicate the direction the arrow is pointing, so their co-operation can be checked before the start. Once again warning the subjects not to touch or move the masks, the room is darkened as much as possible (it does not need to be *total* darkness) and the shutter closed in the first head mask (using a red torch bulb if need be from now on). The examiner continues to close a shutter every 5 minutes in the subjects' masks. At the end of 40 minutes, beginning, of course, with the first subject, the adaptometer test is carried out, the results being recorded by an assistant. Thus, if you have 8 head masks, the shutters of each being closed at 5 minute intervals, 8 subjects can have the minimal light and visual acuity thresholds measured in 1 hour 20 minutes. In the case of small children between 8 and 11 they may be unreliable witnesses in measuring the minimal light threshold, but they are perfectly reliable when measuring the visual perception in a dark adapted eye, and this by itself, by extrapolation from graphs, can be helpful in indicating deficiency in vitamin A.

The most dense stationary filter (0) is used with the wedge, the latter being moved from 0 to 65 on the scale. If nothing is seen the wedge is moved back to 0 and the next most dense stationary filter (1) is used, and likewise for the third stationary filter position (2). Thus the scores run from 000 to 265, each figure corresponding to a unit of brightness. There is a correcting factor for the decay of brightness of the tritium gas bulb, which constitutes the built-in light source. The brightness fades almost in a straight line over 5 years. The values are read off tables for each year of life of the 'tritium gas' light source ('beta' light).

Colour intensity comparison discs

The largest red disc in a set of Traquair targets makes an ideal target for the alternate eye colour intensity comparison test. The eyes are alternately covered and the patient asked if the colour seen is equally bright, or equally red, in the two. Conduction defects of the optic nerve (as in retrobulbar neuritis) typically reduce colour perception; this defect may even precede reduction in visual acuity; it is believed to be due to diminished conduction along the cone system nerve fibres. Lesions of the fundus, even central lesions, on the other hand, that reduce visual acuity, do not grossly interfere with colour discrimination. By evaluation of the fundus appearance and the response, this simple test can confirm a suspicion of an optic nerve lesion.

Other essential instruments

Tonometer

In the absence of facilities for applanation tonometry, the Schiotz or Perkins hand tonometers are excellent instruments. The first should be regularly maintained, so it is worth while taking two.

Loupe

A binocular prismatic head loupe (such as the 'Bin-

omag') is a very useful thing to have, particularly for minor treatments or surgery.

Lid retractors

Various sizes of spring specula are useful for keeping the eyes of nervous patients open for essential examinations, apart altogether from their importance in treatment of a painful eye, such as cauterisation of an ulcer or the removal of a foreign body. Hand retractors, both small and large, to open swollen lids, where the cornea must be examined, are essential, especially in the case of children.

Letters 'C' for vision testing

A wooden letter 'C', painted black, similar in size to the 6/60 letter on Snellen's charts, and charts made up of 'Cs' to correspond, are necessary for recording visual acuity, as is a metre tape.

Binocular microscope

A binocular microscope with a moving stage is necessary for laboratory work.

Gonioscope

The single-mirror gonioscope is used to examine the drainage angle of the eye. The technique is known as gonioscopy. There are two different classifications of the width of the angle. In Scheie's classification we are concerned with assessing the degree of narrowing from 'Wide' to 'Closed'. There are three intermediate positions (Plate 1).

The most popular diagnostic contact lens used (Goldmann's) has a mirror incorporated, which not only transmits the emergent rays from the filtration angle to the observer, but magnifies the picture. A drop of local anaesthetic is placed in the eye and the convexity of the gonioscope then filled with methyl cellulose 1 or 2 per cent before being applied to the cornea. The mirror is best positioned at 12 o'clock on the cornea, which reveals the angle at 6 o'clock. Rotation between the forefinger and thumb enables the average width of the angle to be revealed. At 12 o'clock the angle is most narrow, becoming increasingly wide in an outward direction. Thus, if

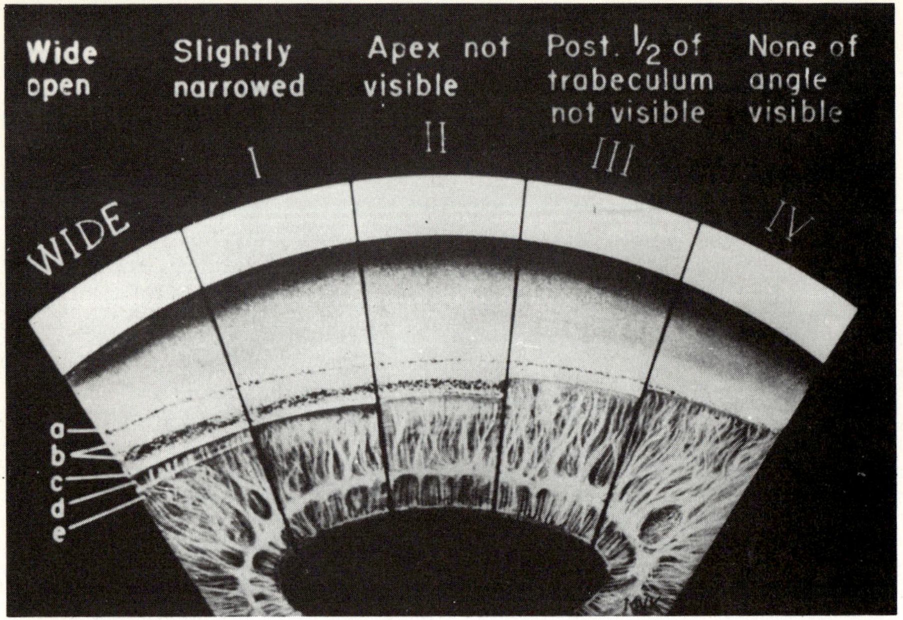

Plate 1 Filtration angle: a. Schwalbe's line; b. anterior and posterior trabeculae (in pigmented eyes the anterior spaces are pigmented as well as the posterior); c. tissue separating Canal of Schlemm from the angle of the eye; d. apex of angle (ciliary body) and e, root of iris

the mirror is placed below at 6 o'clock, a false impression is given as to angle size.

SUGGESTED EYE DROPS, OINTMENTS AND DRUGS

The range of drops and ointments is vast, and unfortunately most are costly. They act efficiently on the anterior half of the eye. Here is a list only of those considered essential and least costly. If alternative drugs are mentioned, that are more costly, they are mentioned for the sake of completeness, in order to save eyes in special cases when they are apparently not responding to any of the more familiar drugs. Several of these drugs can be obtained either as a drop or an ointment. The drop can be given as a subconjunctival injection. In general, ointments are more practical, especially with children, having a more prolonged action and being easier to insert. However, a snag exists: ointments become fluid at high temperatures. In consequence, the economical application of ointments is hard to control in the tropics, for a tube of 'fluid' ointment allows fewer treatments than a bottle of drops.

Mydriatics and cycloplegics

Atropine sulphate 1 per cent drop or ointment. Long-acting mydriatic and cycloplegic for use in keratitis, uveitis and postoperative care.

Homatropine hydrobromide 2 to 4 per cent drop. A mydriatic and cycloplegic with more rapid action and shorter lasting than atropine.

Phenylephrine hydrochloride 10 per cent drop. Direct action sympathomimetic, a mydriatic often used in conjunction with homatropine, gives better and more rapid mydriasis of the negroid pupil than the other alone, and is also short-lasting.

Subconjunctival mydricaine No. 2. Atropine sulphate 1 mg, procaine hydrochloride 6 mg, adrenaline 1/1000 0.12 ml. For rapid dilation of pupil in acute anterior uveitis where posterior adhesions have to be broken down.

Tropicamide 0.5 per cent drop. A parasympatholytic mydriatic and cycloplegic with a rapid action and a minimal effect on accommodation.

Glaucoma

Pilocarpine nitrate 1 to 4 per cent drop for narrow and wide angle glaucoma and to reverse mydriasis.

Acetazolamide 250 to 500 mg tablet. In slow release 'sustets' (500 mg at night) or tablets (250 mg once or twice daily), being an adjunct to pilocarpine treatment in all forms of glaucoma. Each is given with potassium chloride 600 mg to remedy potassium depletion. Diamox can produce crystalluria if used too long.

Ethyl alcohol. In absolute glaucoma, pain can only be eliminated by ocular excision or a retrobulbar injection of from 70 to 90 per cent ethyl alcohol, preceded by a retrobulbar anaesthetic.

Timolol is too expensive at the moment for tropical use.

Special ophthalmic procedures

Lignocaine hydrochloride 2 per cent retrobulbar injection. Anaesthesia of the cornea and conjunctiva for ophthalmic treatment or minor surgery.

Amethocaine hydrochloride 1 per cent topical drop. Good surface anaesthesia.

Oxybuprocaine hydrochloride 0.4 per cent drop. Alternative to amethocaine. Less irritating.

Fluorescein sodium 2 per cent drop or filter paper strip. Diagnostic stain for diseased corneal stroma. Must be washed out well after 45 seconds to give true picture. It is also used in applanation tonometry, where available.

Rose bengal 1 per cent drop. Diagnostic stain for devitalised epithelial cells of cornea and conjunctiva. Not to be washed off.

Anti-inflammatory and allergy preparations

Prednisolone sodium phosphate 0.5 per cent drop or ointment (with or without neomycin sulphate 0.5 per cent as antibiotic accessory). Ocular inflammatory conditions of the eye, both non-infected and infected. Contains no fluorine. There is a danger of inducing glaucoma in susceptible patients if steroids are used a lot. If used too long, those with a fluorine molecule can induce neovascularisation of the cornea; steroids should never be used in an undiagnosed keratitis, unless stromal, rarely in herpes simplex corneal infections; it can predispose to fungus infection.

Betamethasone sodium phosphate 0.1 per cent drop or ointment. As prednisolone above, but more penetrable and contains fluorine.

Oxyphenbutazone 10 per cent (with or without chloramphenicol 1 per cent as antibiotic) drop or ointment. Also as a 100 mg tablet. Ocular inflammation, non-infected or infected, especially if collagen disease is known or suspected.

Xylometazoline hydrochloride 0.05 per cent drop with Antazoline sulphate 0.5 per cent drop. Allergic ocular conditions, but can be quite sensitising themselves.

Anti-infectives

Chloramphenicol 0.5 to 1 per cent drop or ointment. Infections of anterior segment of eye, the first choice for most bacterial ocular infections, including trachoma and all Gram-positive bacilli.

Sulphacetamide sodium 10 to 30 per cent drop or ointment. Infections of anterior segment of eye, including trachoma.

Gentamycin drops. Effective against Gram-negative bacilli.

Natamycin 1 to 4 per cent drop. Fungicidal eyedrop.

Sulphadimidine 500 mg tablet. Trachoma, meningococcal meningitis, bacillary dysentery and pneumococcal pneumonia.

Ampicillin 250 mg capsule. General antibiotic (except against staphylococci), useful for most Gram-positive and negative infections involving conjunctiva, lids and orbit.

Oxytetracycline 100 mg or 250 mg capsule. Oxytetracycline-sensitive infections such as those killed by ampicillin, should be avoided in babies and children.

Soluble penicillin G Sodium 1 mega unit (powder in vials). Penicillin-sensitive infections of eye and lids.

Paediatric suspension of Septrin (trimethoprim 40 mg with sulphamethoxazole (cotrimoxazole) 200 mg. For trachoma and gonorrhoeal infections of eye.

Erythromycin stearate 250 mg or 500 mg tablets. An outstandingly safe, cheap, underused antibiotic, active against most strains of staphylococci and against streptococci.

Flucloxacillin sodium 250 mg capsule. First line drug for treating suspected staphylococcal infections of lid and orbit.

Flucytosine 500 mg tablet. Proven antifungal

against cryptococcosis and moniliasis.

Anti-herpes simplex virus. Tincture of iodine or phenol cautery is the cheapest form of treatment (see text).

Vitamins

Vitamin A 50 000 i.u. capsule or tablet. Asthenia, xerophthalmia, keratomalacia.

Vitamin B (thiamine, riboflavin, nicotinamide and pyridoxine—any preparation) tablet or injection. Vitamin B complex deficiencies including optic neuritis with peripheral neuropathy. Marmite and yeast tablets are alternatives.

Hydroxocobalamin 250 to 1000 μg/ml injections. Pernicious anaemia (and other B12 responsive macrocytic anaemias), tobacco amblyopia, Leber's optic atrophy and toxic optic atrophies of unknown origin.

Some form of iron and folic acid should also be available.

Ferrous sulphate, as tablet, 200 mg t.d.s. For iron deficiency.

Folic acid tablets, 100 μg. 500 μg and 5 mg once daily. For folic acid deficiency

Both vitamin B12 and folic acid are present in the normal diet of man. A deficiency of either leads to a megaloblastic anaemia; in developing countries folic acid deficiency is the cause of most cases of anaemia. Addisonian anaemia is rare. It should be remembered, however, that although the great majority of megaloblastic anaemias have a macrocytic peripheral blood picture, occasionally the red cells are normocytic, or even microcytic, usually when there is a deficiency of iron, which is common, so iron should be given in addition to folate in the tropics. A normoblastic macrocytic anaemia in the absence of megaloblasts is found associated with protein energy malnutrition (PEM), again common in developing countries, and is *un*influenced by either vitamin B12 or folic acid therapy. The underlying disease should be alleviated by pushing protein in the form, for example, of soya bean flour, or leaf protein if available.

The clinical manifestations of vitamin B12 and folic acid deficiencies differ in the absence (usually) of peripheral neuritis and subacute combined degeneration of the cord in the latter. Thus it is unavailing to use folic acid to treat a megaloblastic anaemia in the presence of nervous system lesions; the glossitis may heal and the peripheral blood picture return to normal, but not the nervous system. In consequence, without the back up of a reasonable haematology laboratory, especially where polyavitaminosis is common, the clinician working on his own must have iron, folic acid and cyanocobalamin (in the form of hydroxocobalamin) available, and be prepared to treat his cases empirically.

2

Preparatory information

Visiting the Tropics for the first time—perhaps to be stationed 'up country' in a small hospital with a small laboratory and limited resources—it is useful to be given, as here, certain basic information about what lies ahead. It is also useful to be told how the local scene should slot into the global approach to blinding diseases, how one should prepare the ground before starting work in any new region, and in what respects environmental, racial and socioeconomic factors alter the appearance of the eyes compared with the eyes of those who live in temperate climates.

HELPFUL CONVENTIONS

The tropical world

It is important to know what tropical diseases exist in the area in which you work, for the health of the eye frequently reflects disease in the body, and recovery of eye disease from whatever cause can be hampered by systemic disease.

Several hundred million people are affected by tropical diseases, and many more millions are at risk. They affect all ages and several can affect the same individual; as many as nine infections have been found in a single human being. Not all diseases kill, but all of them weaken the individual, reduce his resistance and limit his work-rate. This is why efforts to control his environment and achieve a better socioeconomy (requiring physical strength and mental alertness) are so often slow, or fail.

Malaria, it is well known, is one of the most widespread diseases in the world. In countries such as the Sudan, transmission is so intense that present efforts of control and treatment are totally inade-quate. It is largely responsible for the high child mortality rate in most developing countries. In India, where it has regressed in the past, it is now returning, and WHO in 1977 announced that once again it must be rated as a major, killing, global disease (Leader Stirling, 1977).

Schistosomiasis is another widespread debilitating disease, different species affecting either the intestine or the bladder. As the intermediary host (snails of varying genera) prefer fresh, still water, dams producing artificial lakes and irrigation canals provide ever new sources of infection. The proportion of the population affected around the lake created by the Kainji Dam in North Nigeria doubled in 3 years. In the Nile Delta the belief is that everybody suffers from it. Although this is an exaggeration, it is true that about 40 per cent of the occupants are affected. One form or other is found in most of Africa, Japan, China, South America and the Near and Far East. *Molluscicides* can be highly effective, but where continuity of control is not maintained, reinvasion soon follows.

Filariasis is a third major disease which reduces man's vitality. There are eight known parasites. To give an idea of how widespread filarial diseases can be *Wuchereria bancrofti* and *Brugei malayi,* both transmitted by mosquitoes, infect some 250 million people in China, Africa, India, South East Asia, the Philippines and several other Pacific islands. Another variety, *Loa loa,* is found along the Guinea Coast, down to and including Zaire. The most dreaded filarial disease of all, *Onchocerciasis,* which can lead to blindness, is found in Africa between 15°N and 15°S as well as in Central America. Here, as in malaria, the remedy to date has been to attempt to eliminate the vector, a black fly. An attempt is in the process of being carried out by WHO to achieve this in the territories irrigated by the three Volta Rivers: the fear is always present, nevertheless, that the black fly, as in the case of the mosquito, may become resistant to the larvicides being used. As in the use of molluscicides, failure of continuity of control at any stage in what must be a selective, repetitive program, will lead to re-invasion.

As if these three widespread infections, malaria, schistosomiasis and filariasis, were not enough, there are many other equally debilitating diseases, which are nearly as widespread, such as amoebic dysentery, trypanosomiasis, leprosy, leishmaniasis, tuberculosis, and several varieties of intestinal worm, which can lead to malabsorption and malnutrition.

Over and above, there is in many parts of the tropical world a background of seasonal malnutrition (when supplies run short before the next harvest) which causes much child blindness, especially where there is malabsorption from the intestines. The common bacterial and viral infections of eye and body—which have a global distribution, and which, in the case of the child, often cause death, or if survival occurs, blindness—are ever present, and there are in addition certain inherited diseases of the blood in Negro races which can debilitate, kill or blind, such as the *sickle cell diseases.*

The tropical world, in short, is a hostile world where infections can arise from contagion, food and contaminated water, from mutations, and from failure to avoid vectors, such as biting insects and small mammals, and intermediate hosts with *their* vectors, such as molluscs, birds and mammals. It is against such a background that patients—whose resistance may be lowered by concomitant disease and malnutrition—are found with seriously affected eyes, which heal with difficulty and may reach epidemic proportions. It is not surprising in these circumstances that the incidence of blindness is in general three times worse than in Europe.

Geographic ophthalmology

Tropical and subtropical countries can be classified according to the environment. Sometimes discrepancies in definition occur, giving rise to uncertainty, so if a term is used it must be defined. The point of raising this question at all is to draw attention to the fact that, if the ecology of the zone in which one is working is known, then one can predict to some extent the major eye diseases likely to be present, and just as importantly what eye diseases are *not* likely to be present. The subject of ecology and ophthalmic disease has only become popular in the past 10 years or so under the title of 'geographic opthalmology'. From it the concept of a multi-discipline approach to specific problems has developed, that is with a multi-discipline team, which includes ophthalmologists, parasitologists, geographers, human biologists, socioeconomists, entomologists and so on, the whole team investigating the people and their environment at the same moment.

Long range prediction of eye conditions, depending on terrain classifications alone, unfortunately permits only of generalisations, as the classification

Table 2.1 Association of common eye diseases with environment.

Bioclimatic zone	Major eye disease found in zones in order of severity
1. Desert	Trachoma, xerophthalmia, cataract, some climatic keratopathy
2. Sahel	Trachoma, xerophthalmia, cataract, some climatic keratopathy
3. Sudan savanna	Trachoma, xerophthalmia, cataract, some river blindness
4. Guinea savanna	River blindness, xerophthalmia, cataract, trachoma, some glaucoma
5. Rain Forest	Cataract, river blindness, glaucoma, some trachoma
6. Equatorial Forest	Cataract, river blindness, glaucoma
7. Estuarine and Coastal	Cataract, some glaucoma, some climatic keratopathy, some venereal disease (especially in ports), some trachoma, avitaminosis B

of terrains is something geographers themselves do not find easy. Nevertheless, terrains can generally be grouped into particular classes where they are of the same kind in several important respects; deserts are a good example of this; deserts, although they have sufficient homogeneity to be recognised as deserts, may themselves differ vastly in size and in their constituent components.

The important factors which lead to such variations—not all being interdependent—include climate, surface form, lithology, soil chemistry, seasonality of the rainfall, and vegetation. Geographers use the term 'land division' to describe a single gross land form. From a medico-biological point of view, the best term to use is 'bioclimatic zone'. All the geographical factors mentioned above, which go to make up the land divisions, influence the anatomy and physiology and habits of the insects, reptiles, fish, molluscs, birds and mammals (including man) within these areas. Collectively, these are the factors, the biological, the geographical and the economic, which by and large create the vectors of diseases and the conditions which predispose to their continuance. One can reasonably expect an average 'within zone' variance in such a classification, but in practice Table 2.1 is a useful guide.

The variability of the eye diseases present in estuarine and coastal zones reflects the cosmopolitan nature of the place: here are the ports and the big cities; here, diseases carried by foreigners often first appear; and here, in the big cities one finds real poverty.

Local information

When posted to a town in a new area (new to the doctor) in a developing country (perhaps new to the doctor), or when moving through such a country on a survey, in each place in which you have to work it is wise to arrange as soon as you arrive an informal discussion with those who might be able to advise you about the diseases known to exist there.

If you are joining colleagues or paramedicals who know the area, they are the first ones whose help you should seek. If on the other hand, you are working alone, or with others equally new to the region, then the chief man, his elders, any local paramedical dresser who might work in the area, an interpreter and a school master, are the people you should call

together for a discussion before doing anything else.

A list of systemic diseases known to occur should be prepared with the corresponding native name or names. A consensus view is often required, as not everyone in such gatherings can discriminate between, say, smallpox and chickenpox. If local custom is not offended, a mother or grandmother can be of great help.

The sorts of question one should ask should be, 'When was the last epidemic?', 'What was it?'. The diet and nutrition should always be investigated, seasonal or total deficiencies being noted. Special attention should be given by direct questioning to the existence of native practitioners. Here, for the first time, one can mention eye diseases and ask what plant medicines are used.

Finally, enquire if mobile medical units ever pay a visit. How often? What do they do? Has there ever been any mass treatment? Against what diseases? How often? When was the last visit of such a team? In this way the information collected forewarns of the diseases, untreated and treated, that may have to be faced. Such a meeting is also an extremely good exercise in public relations, for you are asking your colleagues and the local people to help you, in order to help them.

Preventive ophthalmology

An expressive term which increasingly emerged in the 1970s, largely due to the efforts of Nizetic (1975), was 'Public health ophthalmology'. This descriptive phrase is more or less synonymous with 'preventive ophthalmology'. It encompasses epidemiology, vital statistics, training and education of technicians and paramedicals, socioeconomics and the co-ordination in defined populations of research into specific problems. The public health concept would also make itself concerned with the rehabilitation of the blind which has nothing to do with prevention; that is the only dissimilarity. Preventive ophthalmology implies a multi-disciplinary approach at a very high level, a vast staff and a few selected and enormous projects. It is the ultimate in sophisticated, computerised medicine. It is clearly the way to tackle the major blinding problems of the world (such as trachoma, xerophthalmia and onchocerciasis). It will take a long time to succeed, as its protagonists point out, but it must surely succeed in the end. Inevitably more urgent needs exist than can be dealt with or afforded at the one time, and so the onus of selection of top-level priorities must weigh heavily on the World Health Organisation. Whatever it decides will not please everybody. What role, if any, has the front-line 'medic' to play in all this?

Where the primary aim is after all to prevent blindness, it is essential to obtain for reference the accepted 'International Classification of Blinding Diseases', so that correct records may be collected specifically for the use of those working at a higher level. Moreover, interterritorial data can then be compared. Although the average doctor works outside the framework of these huge projects, he never knows when his own small district may not be suddenly incorporated in some vast high-powered scheme; so, in addition to carrying out his traditional role as one who advises, and treats, and cares for, people in his neighbourhood, he should, from the start, carefully record the *prevalence* (and/or incidence), and the *distribution rate,* of blindness as well as the various *degrees of impaired vision caused by each disease.* Such (descriptive) epidemiological data are basic in the prevention of blinding diseases.

The eye doctor, or doctor concerned with treating eyes, must also keep his thoughts constantly directed towards determining causative factors, attempting to correct them if he can by teaching the population what to do, or what not to do, by recording all his findings with care and by passing his ideas on further up the departmental ladder.

There is a great shortage of doctors in developing countries (1 doctor per 5 million people in some places is not an exaggeration). The shortage of eye doctors is much worse! Clearly, if blindness is to be reduced, it cannot all be left to doctors, and so the concept arises of introducing at village level general health practitioners (GHPs), trained to move as needed from village to village. The World Health Organisation considers such people a basic factor in planning national health development. Most developing countries in consequence will be proceeding along these lines, if not already doing so. The targets must be crystal-clear to the GHPs, and should include how in some instances blindness may be prevented. The local doctor concerned with eye diseases has, therefore, a highly important role to play in this set-up. The information in this book should help him to identify priorities and be able to draw the attention of the visiting primary health workers.

The latter will previously have been trained along certain lines in all aspects of health, but modifications are bound to be necessary to fit the ground situation from time to time.

In between the primary rural health care workers and the local doctor exist in many places smaller specialised mobile teams of paramedicals, including ophthalmic, whose task is treatment, selection for surgery at the main hospital, and public health advising.

Mobile health units have existed for a long time, initially in previous British, French and Italian colonial territories and in the Indian subcontinent, and later in Central and South America. However, these teams (as distinct from static bush or forest dispensaries) were directed against one particular disease, or group of diseases (e.g. sleeping sickness), and they frequently had confused priorities, depending on the ideas of the man in charge. Some fine work was done despite this. Blindness, nevertheless, was only too seldom the target, and collection of base-line data was always neglected. In India mobile surgical units tackled the problem of cataract, and trachoma has been treated for a long time in the near and far East by mobile units which have been immensely valuable, but the size of the problem remained unknown.

The Royal Commonwealth Society for the Blind (UK) carried out one of the first exploration surveys into the causes of blindness in Ghana, Nigeria and the Cameroon between 1952 and 1956.* This was the prelude to a great burst of interest in blindness, and mobile units in general multiplied in Afro-Asia and the Americas. Although the priorities had now become clear, integration of efforts to reduce blindness was missing. What was wanted, and is still wanted in most developing countries, is a *costed basic scheme for an integrated eye service for one 'zone',* e.g. a unit incorporating a central hospital, 2 mobile eye teams, 3 eye doctors, 10 ophthalmic auxiliaries, the whole working with primary health care GHPs or dispensers in villages. Inspired by the vision of Michaelson (1968), Israel stressed the need of such an integrated 'eye service'—if not exactly along these lines, close to it.

*The author was appointed its Director.

A BACKGROUND OF CRYPTO-MALNUTRITION

In the preface to the first edition of his book 'Tropical Nutrition' Nicholl (1938) said, 'in the last few years . . . study of the less cogent results of dietary deficiencies has brought to light the prevalence of many signs and symptoms, such as stunted growth and other effects'. Nicholls was pointing out that up to then only extreme conditions which arise from various food deficiencies, such as beriberi, scurvy, pellagra and keratomalacia, had received much notice. In short, he was stressing the importance of looking for signs of border-line malnutrition.

It is well known that malnutrition delays healing and lowers resistance to infection, hence the importance of recognising it, even when it is not extreme. The most pressing problem in developing countries is protein energy malnutrition (PEM), especially in pre-school children. A study of the diets of various races shows that man can adapt to high or low protein diets usually coupled with low and high carbohydrate intake respectively. The former diet is taken by hunters and to a lesser degree pastoral tribes, and the latter by the labouring classes in very densely populated tropical countries, such as those of southern and eastern Asia (Nicholls, revised by Sinclair & Jelliffe, 1961).

Varied diets

Low protein diets are mainly, though not entirely *vegetarian*. Among the many religious beliefs of Asia is one that says no animal life may be taken by man for any purpose. Some Bhuddist and Hindu sects, like the Jains, extend this to the potential life within an egg. Devout followers of these religions practised vegetarianism long before the word was thought of in any part of Europe or America. Unhappily, protein energy malnutrition is probably at its worst in such societies, for the energy intake is low. True vegetarianism is not alway practical, and many so-called vegetarians are lacto-vegetarians, that is they bend the rules, drinking milk and eating butter and cheese. A true vegan, in whose diet all food of animal origin, including eggs and milk, are excluded, is usually deficient in vitamin A, vitamin B12 and protein. Vegetarianism, even if not strict, is in consequence not a good diet for adults during their prime, nor for growing children, nor for women during the child-bearing period.

As an extension of the philosophy underlying vegetarianism, a *fruitarian* diet has become popular in the West. For some it is the 'trendy' thing to do; for others it is an attempt to avoid ill health. In the tropics it is sometimes forced on a community for several months each year. Fruit alone cannot maintain health; fruit and nuts *might;* careful planning is necessary to ensure the diet is safe, for it could be low in protein, fat, certain essential amino acids, some vitamins and minerals (such as iron). At no time and in no way is a fruitarian diet suitable for babies and young children.

Another 'philosophical' diet adopted by cranks in developed countries, but also, unfortunately, seriously practised in Oriental countries by a minority, is the Zen macrobiotic diet (see also p. 17). It evolved in Japan. Based on a philosophy (the Chinese concept of two opposing forces in everything) it consists of 10 graded diets in which brown rice predominates; the consumption of the Zen diets is said to bring a state of well-being, long life and prolonged youth. The most rigid stages of this progressively severe diet must be severely condemned, as there are obvious deficiencies. Immature persons attracted to the Zen philosophy are at added risk as they must avoid medical advice; the diet, they are told, makes it unnecessary! On the contrary, the macrobiotic diets endanger health, and even life.

Borderline cases

Dietary customs are not usually as freakish as the macrobiotic diets. They can be elicited by enquiry. What is hard to uncover is a diet where the energy intake is border-line. In adults the clinical signs of underlying malnutrition may be very slight. There may be no more than stunted growth and weight with some atrophy of the muscles, particularly in the lower legs. More easily recognised signs are oedema of the lower limbs, in particular over the tibias. Excoriation of the lips and angular stomatitis are also quickly spotted, as are staring eyes (indicative of a retrobulbar neuropathy) and a somewhat uncertain gait.

As far as the pre-school child is concerned, the symptoms are usually more dramatic, but the various lesser degrees of malnutrition must be carefully sought. The nutrition of the young child poses special problems in tropical countries owing to the high metabolic needs during the period of rapid growth, and the limited ability to adsorb and digest the full range of foodstuffs, particularly if they are predominantly vegetable. Babies born in deprived communities are underweight, possibly with substandard stores of nutrients and vitamins due to maternal malnutrition during pregnancy. This does not give them a good start. Despite this, mothers lactate well and breast feed successfully for up to a year or more. The danger period occurs between 1 and 3 years of age, when the child becomes a weanling and the diet which substitutes for the successful mother's milk becomes largely carbohydrate. It is too seldom supplemented. These children exhibit a wide range of clinical symptoms as a result of varying degrees of protein and calorie inadequacy. Four overlapping clinical syndromes (which will be described in Ch. 3) can occur:

1. Kwashiokor
2. Mild kwashiorkor
3. Nutritional marasmus
4. Nutritional dwarfing.

Difficulty arises in spotting mild and intermediate forms of these four syndromes.

The concentration of protein in the diet needed by the very young is about twice that needed by adults. The too frequent presence of severe malnutrition in early childhood, nevertheless, does not necessarily indicate that adults, especially men, in these same communities are equally liable to malnutrition. Furthermore, there is no evidence that young children affected by protein deficiency, if they survive, continue in a state of malnutrition during later childhood and adult life, although they will be somewhat shorter in stature and probably lighter in body weight (Wadsworth, 1977). Recovery is usually full, it seems.

The balance of a diet, especially in adults is far more important than the calorie total, for the eyes are not affected in starvation. A hungry peasant farmer, who eats a very small but well balanced diet, when he migrates to a city as a labourer, may no longer have periods of hunger, but by existing on a diet consisting mainly of white bread and jam his physical condition will deteriorate, for the diet is totally unbalanced.

ENVIRONMENTAL EFFECTS ON THE EYE

Protective mechanisms

The protective mechanisms of the eye and its appendages are highly efficient. Various factors, not readily apparent, cause them to malfunction in the tropics.

The extraocular membranes are lubricated by mucus, which is secreted by cells, especially frequent in the conjunctival fornices, temporal and bulbar conjuctiva, and limbus. The mucus fills in the pits of the corneal epithelial papillae (which can best be seen by the electron microscope). The result of this adherence of mucus is a perfectly smooth convex outer corneal surface, over which the tears, held by surface tension, slowly drift from the upper temporal to lower nasal corner of the eye. If, however, the mucus becomes abnormal in consistency, or deficient as it is in certain diseases, such as chronic infective conjunctivitis, iron deficiency, diabetes mellitus, rheumatoid arthritis and so on, it fails to remain adherent to the corneal surface and falls off; when the consistency is abnormal, it may become harder and be picked out of the eye in small pieces with the fingertips, or less hard, collected into flecks, which float in the tears, as seen with the slit lamp. As a result of the absence of true mucus the tears have nothing to which they can adhere, and flow off the cornea increasingly. Despite the presence of tears, the surfaces of the corneal and bulbar conjunctiva, dry for lack of mucus, become irritated, which further increases the flow of tears over the dried surfaces. Many dozens of minute erosions result and can be demonstrated best by placing a drop of Rose Bengal stain in the lower fornix, the condition being called keratoconjunctivitis sicca (KCS) or 'the sicca lesion'. By holding the lids apart the erosions can be better demonstrated as the surface dries off.

If the role of mucus in lubricating the eye and making it lustrous seems more important than that of the tears (as the development of erosions despite the presence of tears suggests), the tears, nevertheless, are important when a foreign body hits or adheres to the cornea. Reflex secretion helps to remove such objects. Moreover, within the tears there is a substance known as lysozyme, which has bactericidal properties.

If the cornea is injured or diseased, reflex lacrimation is an important sign pointing to the possibility of corneal involvement; photophobia when present in addition indicates the corneal lesion is severe.

A final hazard against which the human eye protects itself reasonably well (by an inborn instinct?) is the damaging effect of the sun. Direct gaze is reflexly avoided, but damage from short ultraviolet radiation (SUVR), especially in the range 290 to 310 nanometers (1 nm = 10 Ångstrom units) is less easily avoided. Although the eye is protected from damage by the overhanging eyebrow and orbit and by narrowing the lid aperture to a slit, the cornea is vulnerable to SUVR reflected from a good reflecting surface such as white coral sand, especially if salt-splashed, as well as from snow and ice.

Despite the existence of these different, efficient, protective mechanisms just described, the eye in the tropical world is still frequently damaged by trauma, disease and the sun. What makes diagnosis so complicated is the fact that identical structural damage results from different causes.

Corneal problems

Minute corneal opacities

The conjunctival anatomy is given in page 29. The nature of the mucus and its importance to the external ocular membranes has been stressed above. It is vital, and in eye diseases like trachoma where destruction of the mucus-secreting cells occurs as a complication of the subepithelial pathology, especially in the late stages, corneal changes similar to KCS may be produced.

Corneal erosions and epithelial opacities may be confused. A superficial viral punctate keratitis (SPK) stains very slightly with Rose Bengal, and may be distinguished from KCS with the slit lamp only, when some spots are seen to be subepithelial (never the case in KCS) often without marked conjunctival involvement, whereas in the sicca lesion not only is the lower cornea affected, but the bulbar conjunctiva as well.

In these days where chemicals are used as aerial sprays increasingly in developing countries, severe corneal erosions in an area corresponding to the interpalpebral fissure occasionally result.

In hyperendemic onchocerciasis areas, in young and old alike, mf. volvulus may simulate SPK when first seen by a newcomer to tropical ophthalmology.

They are linear or polyhedral (fluffy) in shape, and are larger, so should not be confused. They never stain with Rose Bengal. The number of opacities seen may range from 1 to 50 in a single cornea and they exist at all levels.

Dark 'holes' in the eyeball

On examining the eyes of pigmented peoples for the first time, two features may be new to the observer. The pigment cells of Langerhans form dark rings around the anterior ciliary branches as they penetrate the sclera and are very much more pronounced in negroid eyes; secondly, the presence of Herbert's pits (ruptured follicles) at the limbus is a puzzling observation in an eye with healed trachoma, unless one is previously warned.

Accidental injuries

In rural areas, where the densities of the population bear no relationship to the industrial scene, peasant farming is common, hunting in the bush is still possible, and trades such as the blacksmith's and the carpenter's are to be found in every region. For this reason the type of injury one finds is sometimes associated with these activities; these include corneal foreign bodies and small penetrating wounds. Abrasions with infection, conjunctival, corneal and scleral lacerations, and corneal foreign bodies, are also common among farmers. When an eye has had a penetrating injury, the development of *leucoma adherens* (a healed white scar, to the posterior surface of which the iris is attached) is a commonplace; the pupil may be eccentric as a result. Minute corneal foreign bodies, due to iron or stone chips, or to pieces of shell or seeds, when removed, usually leave round subepithelial scars, which may be confused with the residua of corneal viral infections (nummular opacities).

Corneal foreign bodies that contain iron invariably leave a rust ring behind, and it is important to remove this as soon as possible. The explosion of a home made 'dane' gun, or wound from a machete or a penetrating stick or branch, are the commonest causes of destruction of the eye, with need for its excision. Motor car, especially lorry, accidents requiring major surgical repair are increasing all over the tropics.

Blunt injuries without rupture of the eye may lead to blood in the anterior chamber (hyphaema) which when large and untreated can cause staining of the posterior corneal endothelium, residual organised clot in the anterior chamber and even a distorted pupil (Plate 2).

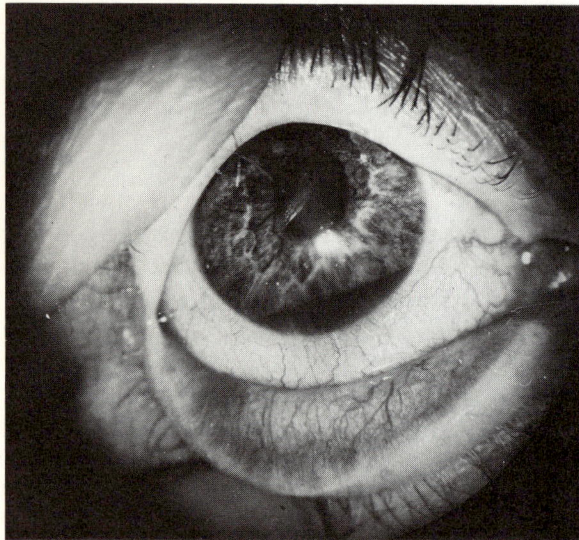

Plate 2 Hyphaema (blood in anterior chamber)

Self-inflicted injuries

Self-inflicted injuries are rare, but may be found among unhappy soldiers, policemen, etc., who want to be discharged. The commonest method of achieving eye damage is briefly to put a seed (such as jequirity, or a little pepper) in the lower fornix. This produces a fiery reaction, followed by a classic scar at 6 o'clock on the bulb, often with a limbal abrasion. The attitude of the patient is one of excessive depression, which is a valuable clue.

Autohaemotherapy

One injury to the external ocular membranes, which occurs despite the various protective mechanisms described above, is when an eye is splashed with alkali or acid, as from a car battery. The best treatment is an old technique known as 'autohaemotherapy', the theoretical basis of which is not certain. It is believed to be based on the hypothesis that in the cornea an enzyme or enzymes are involved in the degradation of damaged collagen and that the inhibitors missing from cornea are present in blood; these inhibitors are made more readily available by juxtaposition. A nonheparinised 2 ml syringe is filled with the patient's own blood, and after a topical anaesthetic has been used and a lid speculum inserted, blood is injected subconjunctivally into the four quadrants until the conjunctiva is lifted up from the underlying Tenon's capsule. Whatever the theory behind this treatment, there is no doubt of its efficacy. Adhesions between the conjunctiva and the underlying tissues are averted, and the cornea becomes lustrous and pain-free overnight. Recent work supports the view that degenerative cornea is self-destructive by liberation from the epithelium of a collagenolytic enzyme, whenever Bowman's membrane has broken down (Slansky, 1970).

Pigmentation of the external eye

Permanent ocular changes occur involving the melanophores in darkly pigmented eyes. The entire limbus in the Negro eye is usually etched with frond-like aggregations of pigment sheathing the capillary loops, quite unlike anything seen in a Caucasian eye, and this has to be taken into account. Invasion of the corneal epithelium with pigment granules is common. Streaks of pigment granules may pass for several millimetres across the surface; whether this phenomenon is posttraumatic or not cannot be said. Sometimes it appears to have no particular origin. There is no doubt that prolonged irritation produces an increased migration of the dense limbal pigment. Chronic irritation due to climate and the presence of hot winds with a high dust particle (like the Harmattan in West Africa and the Arabian Simoom) are probably the main causes of this, especially in the exposed areas of the bulbar conjunctiva. A prolonged period of moderate hypovitaminosis A producing a dry corneal surface is followed by hyperpigmentation at the limbus, which persists after recovery, as does melanosis of the palpebral conjunctiva following trachoma.

The 'measly' eye

Finally, one of the most common and confusing stigmata found is a round, centrally-placed large white corneal scar (leucoma). As mentioned above, this, if unilateral, may follow a wound. Most workers, however, have reached the conclusion that measles in childhood or keratomalacia in the weanling, either singly or together, more often explain the presence of such centrally-placed dense white leucomata than wounds (Plate 3). If the face is pock-marked, one can be fairly certain the cause of the corneal scarring was smallpox. This condition is frequently called incorrectly a 'measly' eye, whatever its nature.

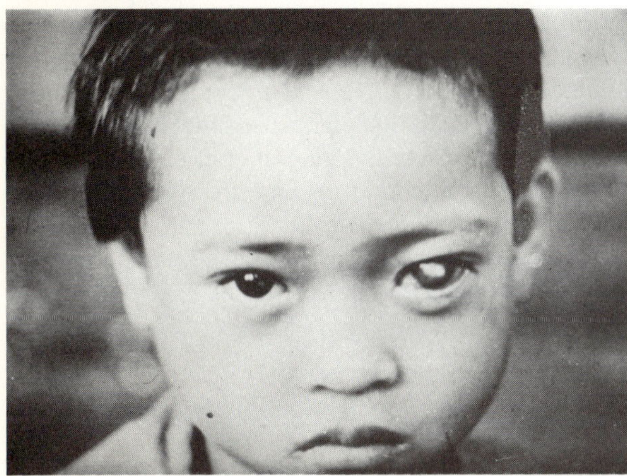

Plate 3 The 'measly' eye: a small scar (leucoma) on the right cornea and a large one on the left, following recovery from measles

Damage due to traditional medical practices

It is helpful to be conscious of the potential graces as well as faults inherent in local medical traditions.

Traditional medicine in India, and to a lesser degree in the Arab world, is in many respects quite as good as the homeopathic brand found in the West, having a certain richness and sophistication derived from many centuries of practice. *Ayurvedic* medicine, essentially Hindu, is approved by the Indian Government, and its practitioners have to train at special government schools for *Ayurveda*. Many sound drugs in use in modern clinics have emerged from these sources, a good example being those derived from the dried roots of the Indian shrub *Rauwolfia serpentina* used by generations of hakims to control the high blood pressures of exasperated Moghul emperors and their Wazirs. Arabic traditional medicine is less appropriate to modern science, being more related to pre-Renaissance

European medicine, but it was seldom harmful and often, as in India, helpful. The Arab malams also developed a special skill (as did the hakims) in dislodging cataracts and restoring sight by *couching*. This is still practised in Afro-Asia: dislocation of the lens is produced by applying external force.

A closely allied system of medicine seen in parts of India, in Bangladesh, Sri Lanka, Burma and Nepal is known as the *Unani-Tibbi* system. Derived from Greek thought and rescued by the Arabs, the basic units of the system are earth, air, fire and water. Plants and minerals are formed by these units, as are animals and man himself, so the mind and spirit of man comes into this variety of traditional medicine to elevate it to the level of the *Ayurvedic* system, although *Unani-Tibbi* developed much later.

The best of traditional Chinese medicine lies somewhere between the Indian-Arab schools and the methods practised today in the more backward of the developing countries. China, too, for a long time had its charlatans, whose main aim was to gull the public for cash. Following the First World War, Ch'en Tu-hsui berated Chinese medicine for its incompatability with modern science: 'Our doctors only talk about the five elements, their production and elimination, heat and cold, *yin* and *yang*, and prescribe medicine according to the old formulae' (Croizier, 1968). Although pre-dated by Egyptian and Babylonian medicine by perhaps a millenium, Chinese medicine has the oldest surviving medical tradition. In the period 3737 to 2697 BC, for example, China produced the first pharmacopoeia in which over 100 drugs are listed. By 100 BC there were 365 drugs, corresponding to the days of our year. The expansion of the materia medica rose steadily thereafter. Perhaps China's greatest contribution towards traditional medical science was the stress they placed on the use of vitamins and the practice of acupuncture. At a time when Hippocrates arrived on the scene (400 BC approx.) and the Greeks had begun to speak about new standards of ethics in medicine, the ancient therapeutic art of acupuncture (the insertion of needles into special points of the body) and moxibustion (the burning of small cones of dried herbs over these same points) had been fully developed in China. In the face of recent evidence of its effectiveness, it cannot even today be dismissed lightly as an outdated exercise.

This brings us to the hard fact that in many

developing countries in the 20th century similar itinerant quacks exist as in ancient times, making a living out of the superstitious peasant. Ghosts, demons, spirits and the supernatural powers attributed to juju are freely quoted to explain physical as well as mental illness—and cures. Instead of joss sticks being tossed in the air as in old China to find the correct prescription, cockerels have their throats cut, because diagnosis of the ailment, and the cure, depends on whether the cockerels end up dead on their backs, their fronts, or their sides after being tossed in the air! Magical rites, a perversion of established religion and a shrewd clinical instinct are interwoven, and sometimes, of course, appear to produce results. What is unforgivable is the 'pharmacopoeia' which the witch doctors use; this is especially true in the case of eye diseases in Africa. Infusions of herbs, leaves, roots and barks are instilled into a painful eye. Sometimes drugs are given in the form of a powder blown into the eyes. Severe pain usually follows with resultant necrosis and scarring. One has no means of knowing whether any of these traditional cures does any good, for only those that harm the eye are seen (Plate 4). Incisions in the upper and lower lids with knives to let out 'poison' are also practised. The adverse results from these various infecting and destructive procedures are seen: ulceration of the cornea, opacification, loss

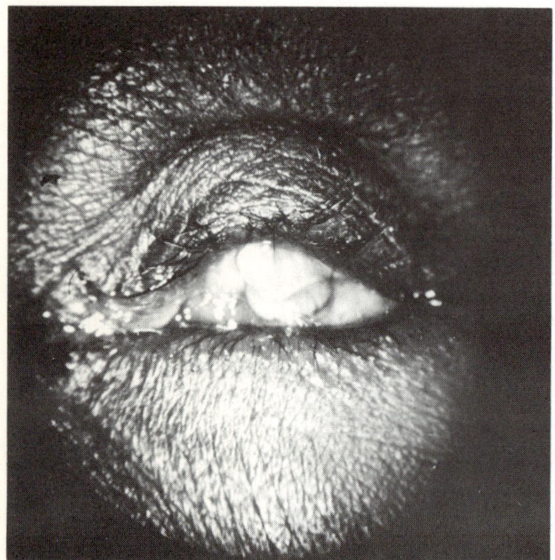

Plate 4 Whatever the original lesion, the eye has been destroyed by the application of native medicine

of the eye, obliteration of the lower fornix, ectropion and phthisis bulbi. If a case presents with any of these conditions superimposed on a known eye disease, then the diagnosis can become baffling in the extreme, and that is why it is important to be aware of their existence.

Drugs to cure diseases other than ocular also sometimes damage sight. For example, the female of the plant *Hagenia abyssinica* ('Kosso' in Ethiopia) is used as an anthelmintic and can cause primary optic atrophy. There may well be other examples of this kind of misjudgement. In one of the lesser-known areas of the world (Papua New Guinea) a phytochemical project has been in operation during the last 7 years. Over 600 plants used for many ailments have been collected. The National Herbarium has been identifying and testing many of them, an excellent example of a developing country looking in a scientific manner for what is good among its own traditional plant medicines.

Damage due to the sun

Climatic keratopathy

Climatic keratopathy is the name given to a condition believed to result from short ultraviolet radiation damage to the cornea. Certainly the evidence is strongly in favour of it (Rodger et al, 1974). It is much commoner than is generally recognised. There have been increasing reports of these specific corneal degenerative changes: first described in the Red Sea and Persian Gulf littoral in the 1930s, more fully in the same region in the 1950s, a few cases were described in Africa, India and Labrador in the 1960s, and in greater detail and abundance thereafter in Western Asia, Arabia and Australia in the 1970s. Without pre-knowledge of the existence of this lesion, many eyes suffering from other diseases are difficult to diagnose. That is why this interesting condition is placed in this particular chapter.

It has already been stressed that the brow and shape of the orbit protect the eye from the direct rays of the sun, and it is also known that dust particles in the air and clouds also scatter direct SUVR. (The absence of cloud over the Red Sea is a feature.) The main source of radiation damage is reflectance of SUVR from good reflecting surfaces upwards into the eye. The best known reflecting surface of the tropics (Rodger et al, 1974) is a salt-splashed white coral beach. On such beaches damage accrues readily where the air is clear of aerosols and there is little shade, especially when economic pressure forces people to work in the open for long periods, particularly likely if there is a cooling wind, as on the shore-line or on an island. Unremitting exposure from childhood onwards is another factor. The largest sand desert in the world—the Rub al-Khali (abode of emptiness)—occupies much of the south of Saudi Arabia; in the east, the Rub al-Khali is a 'sand sea' in which are massive dunes with salt basins (sabkahs), the perfect reflecting surfaces. The author has seen several mild cases of climatic keratopathy in Saudi Arabia among the Bedouin.

It is a complex balance between the different factors mentioned which determines the length of time it takes for climatic keratopathy to develop. Invariably it is a slow process, at least 10 years, so that animals, who do not live as long as man, do not exhibit it. Men working in salt pans or on the seashore are at great risk, for reflectance is great every day. In those that are sporadically affected the change takes a long time to develop and may never develop beyond the first stage.

Climatic keratopathy is a chronic condition. All evidence supports this. The eyelids are puffy; this is particularly noticeable in the case of the lower lids, and is a useful indication of the severity of low-grade persistent SUVR burning (Plate 5). The earliest corneal changes occur in the interpalpebral fissure. Bowman's zone (the surface of the stroma) becomes more dense. This can be seen in the optical section of the slit lamp as a thin grey line, involving the narrow exposed part of the cornea, first commencing at the sides (as does band-shaped keratopathy). With direct illumination, this band, as in band-shaped keratopathy, is interrupted by occasional small, clear, darker areas, round or polyhedral. Later, the entire band will become uniformly grey, without any holes being present. Later still, it will become white. With a slit lamp the altered texture of the zone of discontinuity afforded by structural damage to Bowman's zone acts as a reflecting surface, and by means of this surface, using the techniques of specular reflection and retro-illumination (see p. 4) it can be seen that Bowman's zone has many irregular areas, and the overlying epithelial cells have swollen, the pattern resembling a cobweb or 'veil' more readily visible

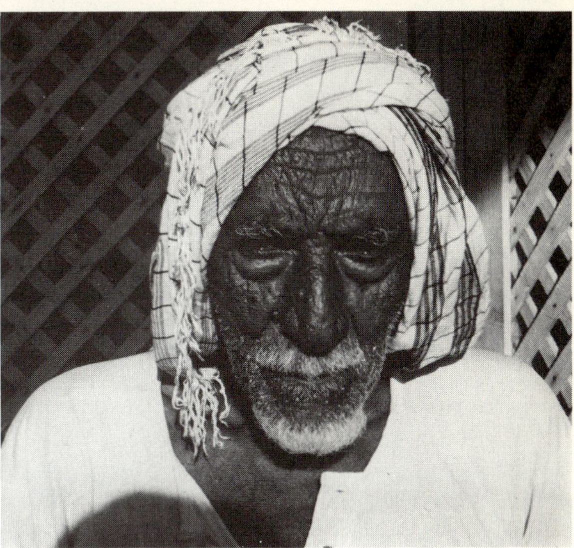

Plate 5 Severe swelling of the lower lids due to excessive and prolonged exposure to SUVR, frequently associated with some degree of climatic keratopathy

than in unaffected eyes. The ready appearance of the 'veil' is a significant confirmatory observation of an early lesion.

When the stromal changes become more severe, the optical section shows increased condensation; the whiter the anterior line of the stroma becomes, the easier it is to see the epithelial 'veil'. At the same time, minute globules (cysts or nodules) begin to appear between the 'tear' and 'anterior stroma' lines, that is within the epithelium. At first clear (cysts), ultimately with light brown coloured solid centres (globules or nodules), these minute structures are most commonly found on the most exposed area of the cornea, i.e. on the temporal side, and increase in size until easily seen by the naked eye. They may spread right across the central area between the lids. This is the classic picture of climatic keratopathy, and at this stage, one should not be in any doubt as to the diagnosis. In the end, the cysts burst; the stromal changes increase; corneal anaesthesia develops; the lids open wider as central vision is obstructed, so the area affected increases, and in the end an elliptical white scar causes total blindness. The pre- and postcystic changes are not as dramatic, and that is probably why so many cases have been missed, and are still being missed. The important thing to note is the age of the patient, the position of any suspicious lesion conforming to the shape of the interpalpebral fissure, the absence or presence of developing cysts, and the ecological background (Fig 2.1 and Plate 6).

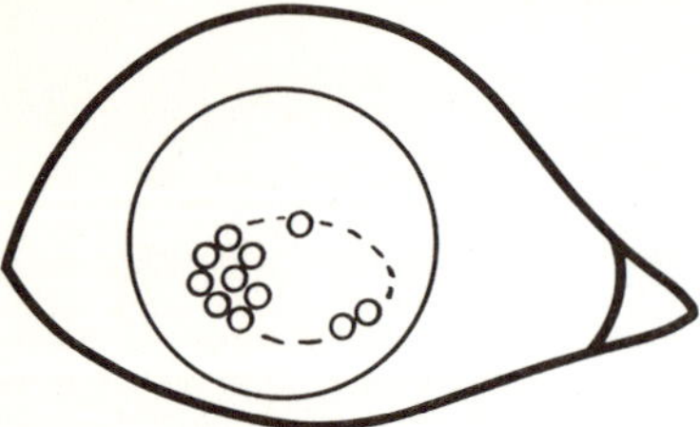

Fig. 2.1 Classic area of cornea affected in climatic keratopathy when moderately advanced with several cysts at the outer aspect

Corneal ulceration is not, as a rule, found. However, in the later stages, when the free endings of the sensory nerves in the cornea have been destroyed and the affected elliptical scar is totally insensitive, foreign material such as sand or even bits of shell (in divers) can lead to painless corneal abrasions and ulceration.

The obvious treatment is to advise the wearing of sunglasses to exclude SUVR. Debridgement of the cysts, especially when the stromal change has not progressed too far, greatly helps in renewing visual acuity.

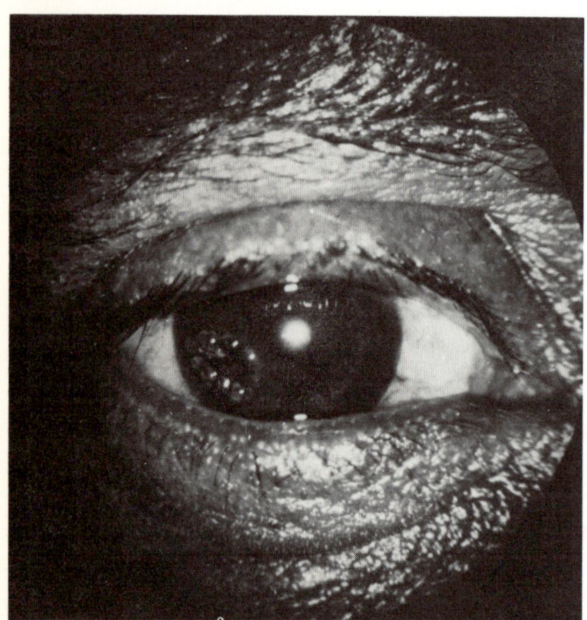

Plate 6 Climatic keratopathy, cystic stage

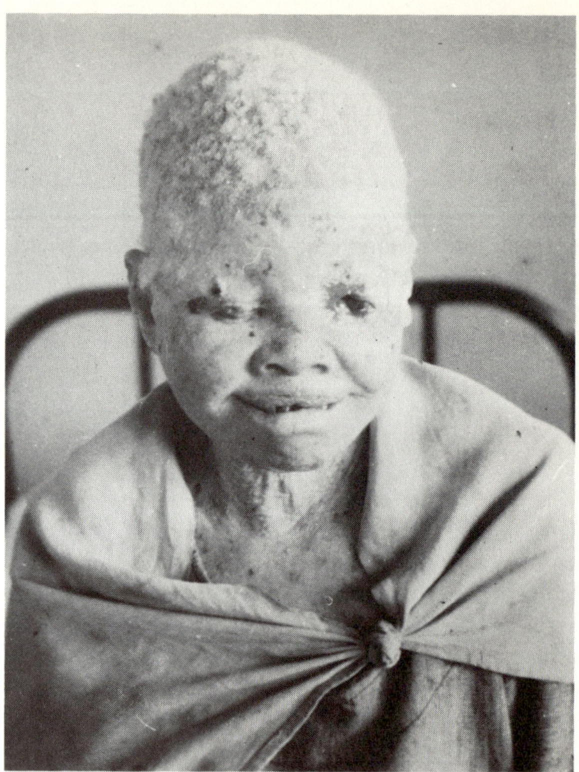

Plate 7 Albinism in an African with polymorphic light eruptions and corneal changes

In albinos (Plate 7), life can be unbearable, especially when light sensitive.

Acute SUVR keratopathy

Whereas the condition known as 'climatic keratopathy' takes a long time to develop, presumably because it is a result of the summation of SUVR low-grade burning, an acute SUVR keratopathy can result in the short term where the dosage and exposure are maximal. As has been seen, it is the rays reflected from the ground which do most damage, and so the nature of the ground is important. Salt or salt splashes on white coral sand, ice (as in the Labrador ice packs), or snow, afford the best surfaces for reflectance, and can damage unguarded eyes even when the subject is sitting under an umbrella; the clarity of the air also plays an important part. Next to no SUVR reflectance occurs from earth or brown sand or grass, and none is reflected from water despite popular opinion to the contrary. The bulk of

SUVR striking water passes directly into it, although at a very oblique angle of incidence minor reflectance does occur.

At high altitudes, where the clarity of the air is well known, and snow commonplace, reflectance from the snow's surface is so great that an acute keratopathy (snow blindness) will inevitably result if the eyes are unguarded. Eskimos and Lapps wear fine leather head bands with pin-holes over their eyes to guard against snow blindness and counteract any refractive error. Acute keratopathy has been noted in the eyes of Red Sea Islanders, who sit day after day on salt-splashed sand spits, watching fish traps (Rodger, 1973). Industrial sources of SUVR (arc welding, oxyacetylene, etc.) produce the same clinical symptoms if protective goggles are not worn. Acute SUVR keratopathy from industrial sources or in alpine resorts is easy enough to diagnose, but is not likely to come into the reckoning if seen in an inhabitant of a tropical island!

The acute lesion, unlike the chronic, is an epithelial change only. No permanent damage results unless the condition which produces it is repetitive. The symptoms are those of any acute corneal lesion: photophobia, lacrimation, blepharospasm and acute pain. Oedema and redness of the lids are usually also present. When stained with Rose Bengal the corneal epithelium is seen to be irregularly swollen, with several erosions in the pits and hillocks of the oedematous front face.

Two or three treatments with a weak topical anaesthetic, spaced out, with or without the addition of a weak adrenaline eyedrop (which has the additional value of paralysing the pupil temporarily and interrupting ciliary neuralgia) will keep the patient comfortable until the effects of the burn wear off, usually within 8 hours. Treatment of this nature should not be prolonged, as severe corneal damage can result from excessive use of topical cocaine-derivative eyedrops.

Macular burning

Man, as stated earlier, avoids staring at the sun. The optical system of the eye acts like a burning glass, so that a steady gaze at the sun can burn a hole in the retina. It is well known that in the absence of protective glasses the sudden intense light of the sun, when it reappears at the end of an eclipse, can produce such macular burns in those whose interest is so intense that they forget to avoid the sun's rays. Mentally disturbed patients have been reported several times with macular burns.

The early ophthalmoscopic appearance is one of perimacular oedema; later, either a macular hole becomes visible, or the macular area exhibits a few small pigmented particles. In either case central vision is grossly affected. Where the hole is deep (the punched out hole of 'eclipse blindness'), then defective sight is permanent. These are the classic appearances of macular burning, for which, unfortunately, there is no treatment. Use of trichromatic filters in an ophthalmoscope helps in diagnosis.

It must be obvious from all that has been written in this chapter that the newcomer to ophthalmic problems in the tropics, especially if he is also a newcomer to the tropics, has a great deal more to consider than his counterpart in the West. The only comfort he has is that many of the most common blinding diseases in the West are rare in developing countries.

3

The major blinding diseases in the tropics

In developing countries, for the greater part tropical, the diseases which are most responsible for suffering and for the greatest incidences of blindness are cataract, trachoma, xerophthalmia, and river blindness (which is geographically restricted, or it would be the greatest menace of all); in addition to these four diseases there is another one, leprosy, in which the proportion of blindness is not known. It appears to be high, but as the millions of lepers in the world for the greater part live isolated, rejected existences, it is impossible to be sure.

In this chapter these diseases—with the exception of cataract, which is a surgical problem and only briefly described here—are discussed in great detail because of the unique position they occupy.

CATARACT

Progressive lens opacities may advance in both eyes until the patient is blind. The author has found in most of the villages he has visited in the tropics that about one-third of all blindness is due to this defect, which is known as a *cataract* (Plate 8). The word 'Cataract', meaning a cascade or waterfall, derived in the first instance from Greek, and later—in Roman letters—from Latin, does not give as good a description as the Hindi phrase 'moti pani' (pearl water).

Where surgery is available sight can be restored, but in developing countries many millions of people suffer blindness because of the lack of surgeons. The late Sir Henry Holland recognised this need and instituted the first Eye Camps in India, where by a well organised co-ordinated effort in the cool season on the part of the surgeons, many hundreds of cataract operations are carried out weekly, the patients being nursed in tents by their relatives under supervision. Couching a cataract is still practised in many countries, including the one in which it is believed to have originated, India. It is more commonly practised today in Africa. From India the technique reached Alexandria and some time later Egyptian migrations southwards of Hamitic people (mainly the Fulahs) brought couching as far as West Africa. Itinerant Hausa 'malams' made quite a living out of it.

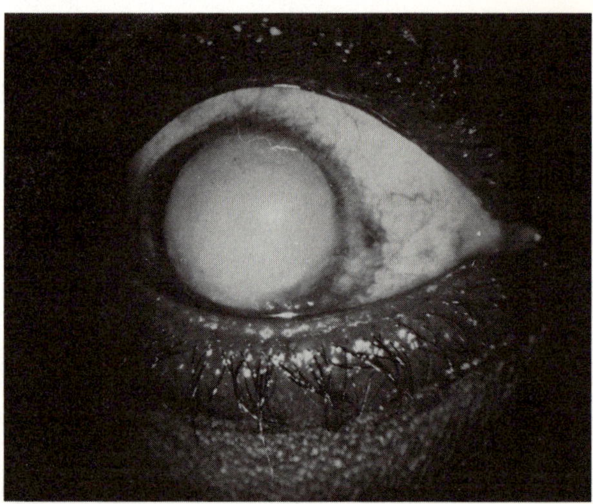

Plate 8 Mature senile cataract having dislocated into the anterior chamber

The Indian method consists of puncturing the sclera behind the root of the iris and with a blunt spud pushing the lens downwards, into the posterior chamber. In Africa a long acacia thorn is burned in fire until it is as hard as steel; the malam squats before his patient (also squatting, his head held); he places the thorn in the correct position; he then knocks the thorn sharply downwards and backwards, dislodging the cataract and clearing the pupil. Usually the capsule has only a single small hole and lens matter does not escape. If it does, uveitis (or endophthalmitis) is the likely outcome. The author has several times seen cataractous lenses lying in the bottom of the posterior chamber, many years after couching, in perfectly quiet eyes.

As cataract is a surgical problem, it need not be discussed in detail here. In essence, the internal metabolism of the human lens has altered when opacities show. It is an ageing process, hence the term senile cataracts, an involutionary change, which occurs to some degree in the majority of eyes. The metabolism of the lens is also affected when the surrounding structures are inflamed, or in endocrinal disorders (secondary or complicated cataracts), or when the lens capsule is broken (traumatic cataract). Inflammatory exudate from the iris sometimes conceals a complicated cataract.

Finally, cataract is also found as a congenital phenomenon all over the world.

The opacities develop in different ways. With the slit lamp, one can by frontal (direct) illumination and in optical section sort out exactly where the opacification lies. The diagrams (Figs 3.1 to 3.7) show the outlines of the principal types of cataractous change which face the surgeon. The treatment of cataract is described in Galbraith's 'Basic Eye Surgery' (1979).

Viewed with the ophthalmoscope (through a +10 lens) the opacities are seen as dark structures against a red background. With the slit lamp, using direct focal illumination, the opacities are white or yellow, and sometimes even red (brunescent). Coloured crystals (cholesterol) may occasionally be seen, usually along the optic axis in the anterior or posterior cortex or the nucleus. They have apparently no particular significance.

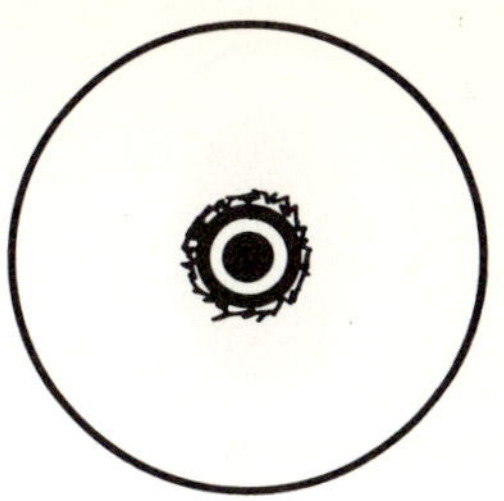

Fig. 3.2 Cataract. Congenital anterior or posterior polar and capsular opacities with reduplications of the rings (ophthalmoscopic view). The depth of the opacities is more easily ascertained with a slit lamp

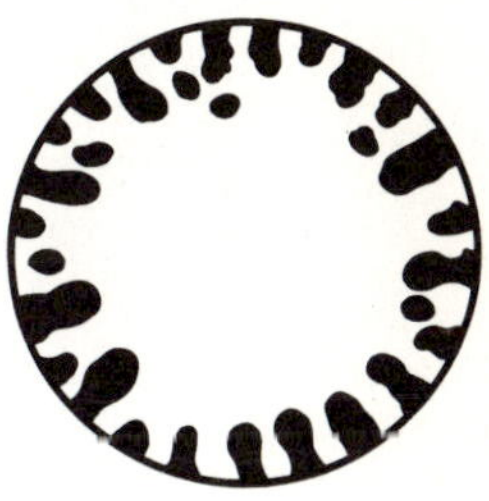

Fig. 3.3 Cataract. Hereditary cortical or 'blue dot' opacities (ophthalmoscopic view)

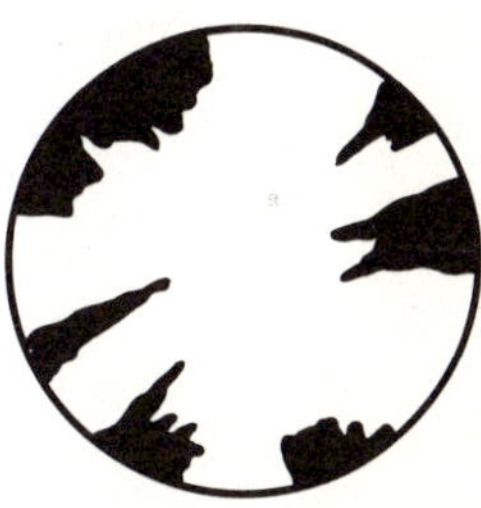

Fig. 3.4 Cataract. Probable shapes of cortical (cuneiform) opacities (ophthalmoscopic view)

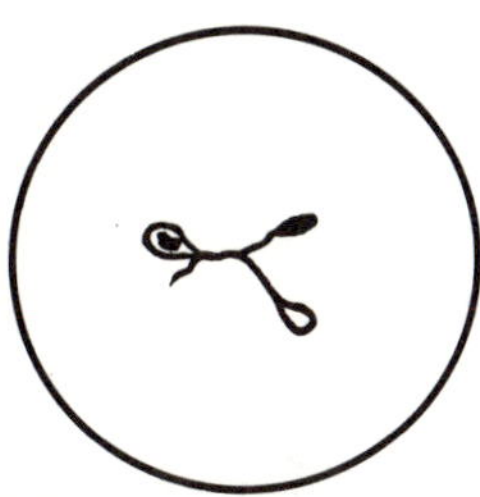

Fig. 3.1 Cataract. Congenital anterior axial or sutural opacities (ophthalmoscopic view)

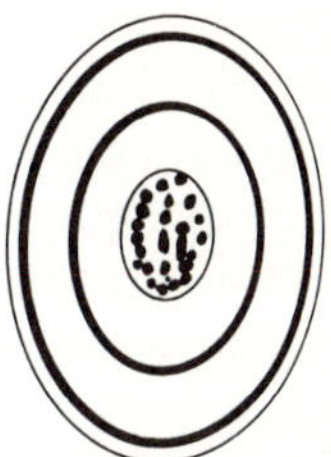

Fig. 3.5 Cataract. Congenital fetal nuclear opacity (slit lamp view)

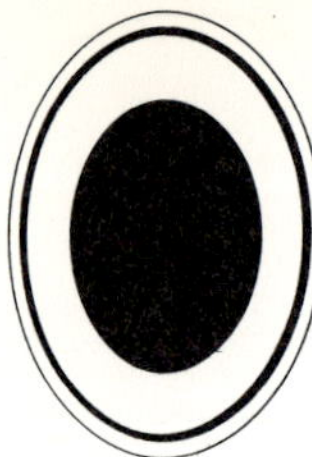

Fig. 3.6 Cataract. Nuclear sclerosis, the most common form of senile cataract (slit lamp view)

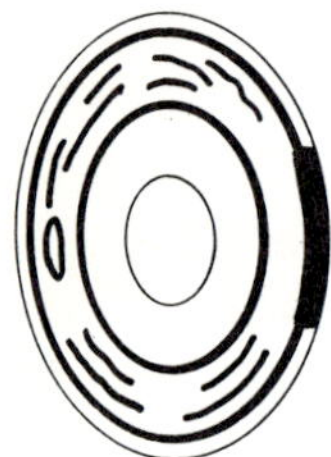

Fig. 3.7 Cataract. Cortical cuneiform opacities with a water cleft in the anterior cortex and a subcapsular (cupuliform) opacity in the posterior cortex. The nucleus is clear (slit lamp view)

TRACHOMA

The natural history of trachoma

The World Health Organisation estimated a few years ago that throughout the world trachoma affects 500 million people, of whom at least 2 million have been totally blinded and many more (millions, one assumes) suffer from defective sight (Tarizzo, 1973). Reports from West Africa show the disease accounts for slightly more than one quarter of blindness from all causes, and yet this disease is preventable. The prevalence of trachoma in India, Pakistan, the Arab world and the Far East is worse than in Africa.

By studying the ecology beforehand one can be alerted to the presence of this disease. A dry climate appears to be an essential element in areas of hyperendemic trachoma. Around the equator, as in Zaire, where there is a heavy, lengthy rainfall and a low density population, there is no endemic trachoma at all, although in all other respects the living conditions should predipose to it. The density of the population is another factor which must always be considered and the socioeconomic factors of the area in which the infection is present also play a part in

perpetuating it. For example, trachoma has been known to affect one half of a town, the half occupied by a poorer, pagan tribe, who cooked amidst dense smoke inside their houses, whereas the other half, that occupied by a richer Moslem tribe with cleaner houses, whose custom it was to cook outside, was comparatively free from the disease. Thus public health factors in addition to climate can affect the spread of the disease in a community and are important targets in its prevention.

Development of the lesions

For a long time trachoma was defined as a keratoconjunctivitis resulting from eye to eye infection with one of the group of large viruses (Chlamydia, formerly Bedsonia), the responsible one being named *Chlamydia trachomatis;* the histopathology was always linked with the presence of certain intracellular microcolonies of this virus described as 'trachoma inclusion conjunctival (or TRIC) agents'. This is for the greater part true wherever endemic trachoma exists, whether it blinds or not. Later, largely through the work of Barrie Jones, which he summarises in Jones (1977), it was discovered that typical cases of trachoma can arise spontaneously by sexual transmission from a genital reservoir (even in a hyperendemic area, if much less commonly) and can be found in the newborn, the child or the adult. Because of the presence of infection in the birth canal, it was not surprising to learn that ocular infections from this source occur not only at birth, but by touch, by contamination of clothing and even in pools where people swim and wash. As some genital mucosal TRIC agent infections are less destructive, they have been designated as 'paratrachomas'.

It is important to note that *Chlamydia trachomatis* includes not only the TRIC agent (trachoma and the paratrachomas) but also the LVG agent (Lymphogranuloma venereum described on page 91), and that there are striking biological differences between these two. The microbiological classification of chlamydial agents relevant to the eye and the diseases they are associated with have been worked out by Jones in 1980. The serotypes of the two agents listed in the table need not concern us here, but the authoritative scope of Jones' findings makes it certain that this classification will come into universal use (Table 3.1).

Table 3.1 Interrelations of chlamydial organisms and serotypes (Jones, B. R. 1980. Trans. Ophthal. Soc. U.K.)

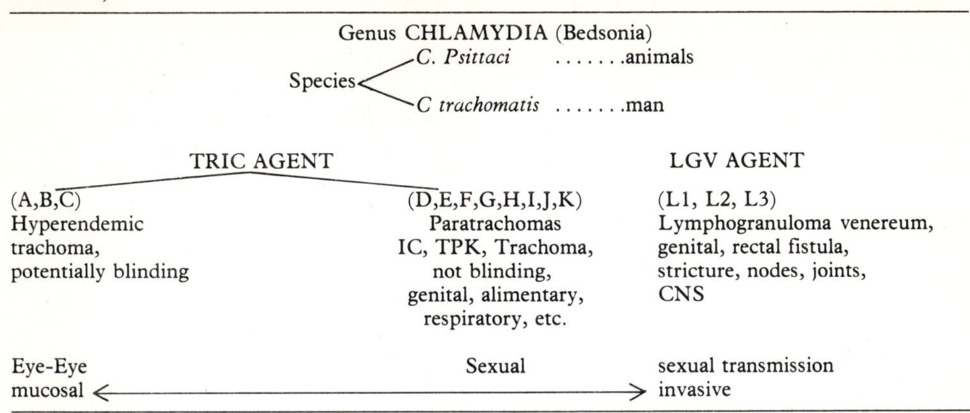

To sum up Jones has put it this way: in the vast majority of cases infection (with the TRIC agent) is transmitted from person to person by intimate sexual contact involving at various times genital, rectal, oral or other mucosal surfaces. No doubt it can be directly transferred to the eye during such activities. However, in the vast majority of cases it appears to be transferred to a genital mucosal area, and then by means of transferring a genital discharge by hand, or other vectors, it reaches the eye.

Trachoma is found in nearly all tropical countries as well as in parts of Europe in those areas where the public health structure has not yet been made adequate for the needs of the people. Within hyperendemic areas the effective reservoir for transmission is in the eyes of those with active trachomatous secretion, babies and young adults alike suffering; the younger the child, the more likely is there to be an infective eye discharge. Transmission occurs by direct touch, from infected clothes and bedding, and by eye-seeking flies, which convey infection because before feeding on the ocular secretions of a new subject they vomit up the previous (infected) meal. In short, hyperendemic trachoma is most common where there is poverty, dirt and overcrowding; it is to be found at its worst when there are ocular irritants as from smoke in huts in which a fire is burned for cooking, or for warmth, without an adequate chimney (as indicated earlier), where the climate is hot and dry, and where winds and dust are the rule. Secondary bacterial and repeated TRIC agent reinfections greatly affect the severity and course of the disease. One other factor which seems to be closely related to the worst ocular complications of trachoma is a seasonal outbreak of bacterial purulent conjunctivitis (Koch-Weeks, pneumococcus, *Staphylococcus aureus* and Moraxella), each attack massively activating *C. trachomatis* infections. This may be related to the peak period of reproduction of the fly population.

Blinding hyperendemic trachoma

The diagnosis is greatly helped if a slit lamp is used (see Ch. 1). MacCallan's classification still holds (MacCallan, 1931), and is given below:

TR I. Stage one is characterised by increasingly diffuse redness of the palpebral conjunctiva lining the upper lids and covering the tarsal plate. On close inspection with some form of magnification the congested conjunctiva is seen to contain many small red dots (papillary hypertrophy); following this appearance much larger pale (lymphoid) follicles in which the virus is actively proliferating coincide. Both these features then spread across the entire upper palpebral conjunctival surface, not just the outer parts. The proportion of papillae to follicles varies.

In this same stage, the acute, the upper part of the cornea becomes oedematous and also infiltrated with inflammatory cells, revealed as a faint grey opacification invading the upper arc of the cornea from the limbus. The advancing margin of the opacification is not necessarily straight edged, more usually irregular. The most superficial vessels at the limbus, the capillary loops, become dilated and elongated, growing down between Bowman's membrane and the epithelium into the grey infiltrate to form the classic *pannus trachomatosus* (Fig. 3.8). In the later stages pannus will appear in the stroma below Bowman's membrane as well. Only rarely does one see pannus in the lower cornea, and then only in conjunction with upper pannus. It is very rare to find the whole limbus involved, but not unknown. It is useful to measure the depth of the pannus from the limbus inwards in mm. The acute stage (TR I) can last from a few months to several years.

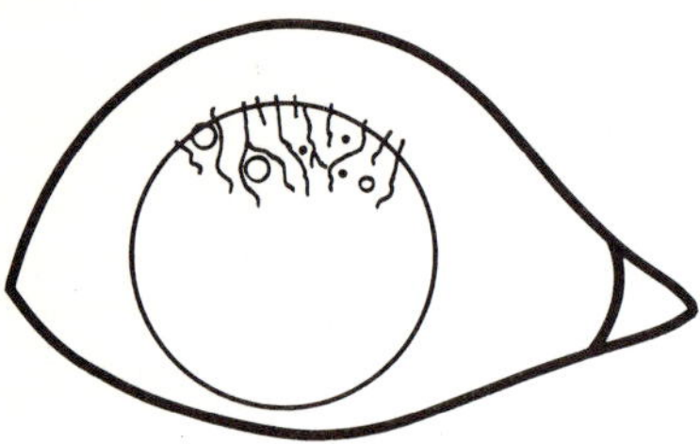

Fig. 3.8 Trachomatous pannus with a few corneal opacities and one large follicle at the limbus (TR II)

TR II. Stage two is still associated with active infection, in which all the signs described in stage one increase, sometimes grossly; it is often called the 'florid' stage for that reason. In this stage the whole upper lid becomes thickened; the papillae enlarge so that the palpebral conjunctiva is very congested. The follicles cannot be missed and have been described as looking like 'sago grains', scattered over the hyper-aemic, red, velvety conjunctiva, and on close inspection on the bulbar conjunctiva down to the limbus (Plate 9). The pannus has now passed towards the apex of the cornea, and here and there may have broken through below Bowman's membrane. Even with the naked eye, the red vessels in the cornea, being dilated, are visible.

In a grossly affected eye at this stage, the appearance may be made worse, and the diagnosis more complicated, by a coexisting spring catarrh (rare), or by a secondary bacterial infection (common). In the latter the secretion will be mucopurulent. When the follicles are large or the reaction gross, in deeply pigmented races melanophores may coat the palpebral conjunctiva with pigment. Even after healing most of the pigmentation remains.

TR III. Stage three is characterised by the onset

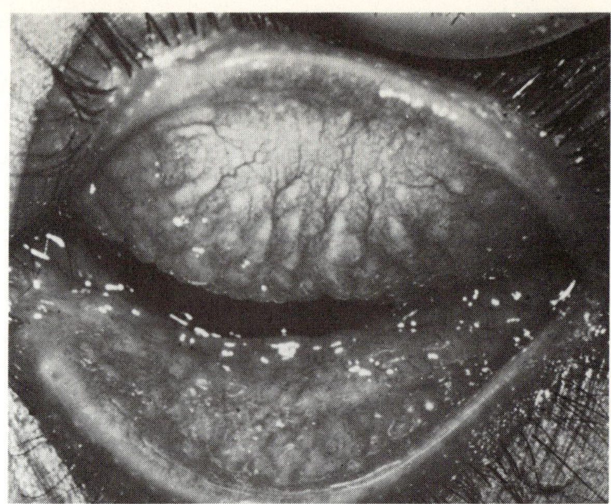

Plate 9 Acute trachoma with follicles and papillae

of healing. The follicles rupture, any at the limbus producing a striking appearance (Herbert's pits). Scar tissue starts to develop most noticeably on the under surface of the upper lids. Strands of scar tissue appear irregularly within and below the conjunctiva, in which there may still be signs of active disease, although less severe. The scars, at first pink (against the red congestion) later become white, like all scars, and deform the soft tissue of the lid down to and including the tarsal plate. Outbreaks of bacterial or a new infection by *Chlamydia trachomatis* at this stage start things all over again; thus stages two and three can co-exist for many years. With repeated acute attacks more and more scar tissue appears and an ever-increasing pannus covers the cornea.

TR IV. In the fourth and last stage, healing has become effected. No inflammatory signs are evident. Papillae and follicles have gone. The scar tissue adopts no particularly specific shape, but the midtarsal area is invariably where it is most striking; it can adopt the shape of small spurs, or sheets, or more rarely a mosaic, outlined by what is left of pink conjunctival tissue. The blood vessels in the pannus hold less blood or are empty. Herbert's pits may be seen along the upper limbus (see TR III).

The disastrous effects of trachomatous scarring consist of deformities of the upper lid and opacification of the cornea (Plates 10, 11, 12).

Thickening of the upper lids in TR III and IV give a hooded appearance to the eyes, a pseudoptosis. Scarring of the upper lids involves the tarsal plate,

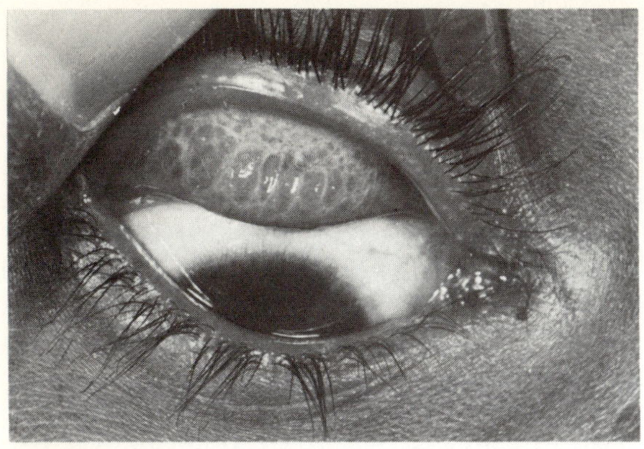

Plate 10 Early conjunctival scarring in trachoma

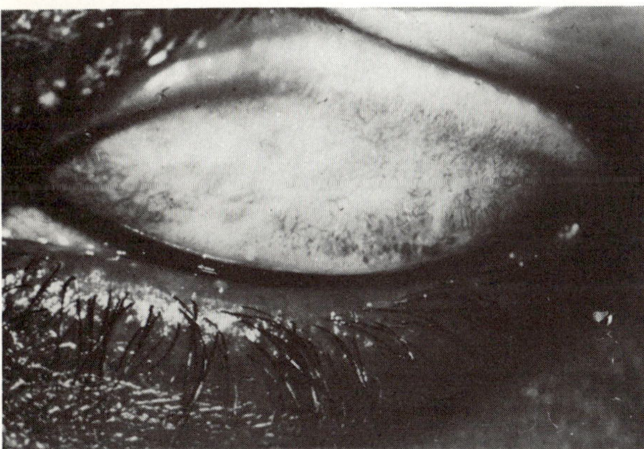

Plate 11 Quiescent trachoma with almost total scarring of palpebral conjunctiva of upper lid

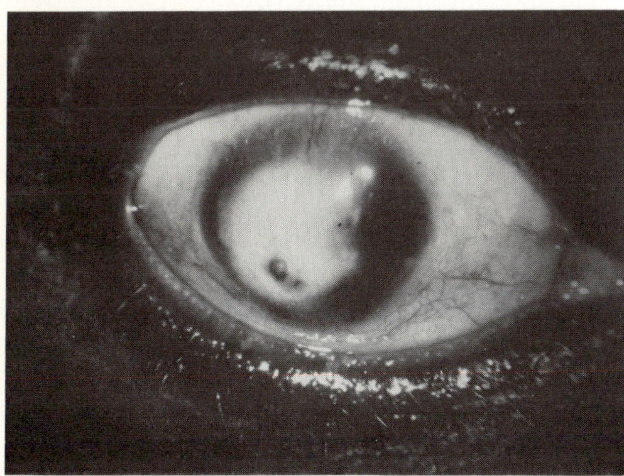

Plate 12 Leucoma adherens following perforated corneal ulceration in trachoma. Note pannus

causing it to buckle and twist and frequently inturn (entropion). In tropical countries one or other or both these features indicate a past trachoma. When entropion exists the lashes in consequence rub on the cornea (trichiasis); this leads to continuous irritation and lacrimation, until the corneal surface itself becomes scarred and anaesthetic. Alternatively, trichiasis in the active stage can break down the corneal epithelium and lead to ulceration. Bacterial infection of ulcers created in this way can lead to loss of eye.

Non-blinding endemic trachoma

This term is of particular value in the epidemiological classification of trachoma in any particular area. It describes those regions where trachoma is mild, either because the factors contributing to severe trachoma are not all present, or are reduced. Such regions are called meso- or hypoendemic trachoma areas. In them, although reduction of vision may be common, blindness due to the complications is minimal. For all that, the pathogenesis is the same in these regions as it is in hyperendemic blinding trachoma regions. The transmission is identical, that is largely eye to eye, and in some by genital transmission as well. Such mild, non-blinding endemic trachoma resembles in many respects the adult paratrachomas.

Treatment

Although sulphonamide eye ointments are effective and cheap, more effective still is one of the tetracycline eye ointments, especially if given with a course of sulphonamides by mouth.

Sulphonamide eye ointment (Albucid 10 per cent) is the treatment of choice in meso- or hypoendemic non-blinding trachoma, given 3 times daily for 1 week at monthly intervals in 2 or 3 treatments.

In a hyperendemic area Achromycin eye ointment (tetracycline hydrochlor. 1 per cent) 4 hourly for 1 week at monthly intervals for 3 treatments is required. Albucid eye ointment (sulphacetamide sodium 10 per cent) is an alternative, but is not so effective. Chloramphenicol eye ointment, potent against so many secondary bacterial infections, is less effective against trachoma.

In all endemic trachoma areas, in addition to topical treatment, as above, sulphamethazine tablets (sulphadimidine 500 mg) should be administered twice daily for 1 week and a second course after a month's rest. In refractory cases, provided the fluid intake is pushed, the daily dosage of sulpha tablets can be doubled. Alternatively, tetracycline 250 mg capsules 4 hourly for 1 week may be given and a second course after a month's rest.

Children are best treated with a suspension of Septrin (sulphamethoxazole 200 mg and trimethoprim 40 mg in 5 ml) as follows:

under 2 years	2.5 ml
2 to 5 years	2.5 to 5 ml
6 to 12 years	5 to 10 ml

twice a day in each case for 1 week, repeated after a month as before.

THE PARATRACHOMAS

Here we are dealing with an initial genital mucosal TRIC infection, which can be passed from eye to eye as well, and produces either a blenorrhoea or a conjunctivitis.

Blenorrhoea of the newborn

Otherwise known as ophthalmia neonatorum, it is important to distinguish this condition, which is less destructive and which results from genital mucosal infection by TRIC agent *C. trachomatis* from the far more serious blenorrhoea due to gonococci or other bacteria such as Koch-Weeks bacillus, *Moraxella, Staphylococcus · aureus* and *Pneumococcus,* all of which can cause purulent ophthalmias. The paratrachoma caused by the TRIC agent may be associated with any of the bacterial infections, and in the tropics this is unfortunately often the case. The most serious condition is probably where the virus and the gonococcus are associated, but fortunately in remote areas of Africa and Asia, this is not common (see p. 74).

Gonococcal ophthalmia has an incubation period in the newborn of only a few days, whereas it takes longer to appear (5 to 15 days) in the case of infection with the TRIC agent. In the purulent ophthalmias due to gonococci or other bacteria, the initial watery discharge quickly turns into a purulent one. The lids become swollen, tense and deeply red, as in an orbital cellulitis. Pus oozes out from between the tightly closed margins. It is impossible to open the eyes without the aid of retractors, and even then so great may be the congestion and oedema that only a glimpse of the apex of the cornea can be obtained. Early haziness of the corneal apex does not necessarily indicate a pending risk of corneal ulceration and perforation, but the risk is there. Even if the eye does not perforate, despite treatment, especially when delayed, a permanent scar will result. Gonococci are increasingly penicillin-resistant, and treatment is no longer as simple as when this antibiotic was first used. Blenorrhoea of the newborn due to the TRIC agent *C. trachomatis,* in the absence of secondary infections, is less severe; it may even only affect one eye. The secretion is mucopurulent as in gonorrhoea. The lids are also initially grossly swollen and oedematous, but they are less tense and red. Without treatment, it can regress. Follicles can be seen on both upper and lower palpebral conjunctivas in from 6 to 8 weeks, yet the cornea is not grossly affected. Staining the secretion and scrapings from the conjunctiva with Giemsa as a diagnostic aid is important. More important still with an infant is to start treatment as early as possible, and to take no chances by giving a wide spectrum of antibiotics.

Treatment—to embrace all eventualities—is carried out *hourly* for 2 to 3 days using Achromycin eye ointment with chloramphenicol 0.5 per cent eye drops. Such treatment may have to be combined with oral Septrin, either as a syrup or suspension (half doses for small children), twice a day for 1 week. A mydriatic such as Atropine 1 per cent should be used as well as a safeguard (see Ch. 1 for details of drugs).

Inclusion conjunctivitis

This variety of paratrachoma due to infection by the TRIC agent has an acute onset in a child, adolescent or adult. A watery eye soon discharges mucopus; the eye is red and very irritable; large follicles arise usually in the lower fornix after about a week. If in the upper lid conjunctiva, the midtarsal area usually escapes. There are no serious complications, but it causes extreme discomfort, perhaps for several months. In the late stages when the eye is no longer red, the follicles may still be present, and will only slowly disappear. Secondary infection in such susceptible conjunctival tissue can always occur, leading to a more intense purulent ophthalmia.

The condition is best treated as a hypoendemic non-blinding trachoma, but tetracycline may be substituted for Albucid if the condition is refractory.

Inclusion punctate keratoconjunctivitis

The last of the paratrachomas to be described is the TRIC virus punctate keratoconjunctivitis, which lies in an intermediate position between a non-blinding hypoendemic trachoma and inclusion conjunctivitis. It looks exactly like the latter condition with the addition of epithelial and (later) subepithelial superficial punctate keratitis (SPK) *but no pannus.* The infection, acquired initially from the genital canal, spreads indirectly or by eye to eye transmission, as in the case of inclusion conjunctivitis. In addition to redness and watering and a mucopurulent discharge, there is photophobia by reason of the corneal involvement. The SPK can persist for a long time (up to a year) unless vigorously treated at the start, and even then the corneal opacities may remain in both children and adults for many months. The absence of pannus and conjunctival scarring is the only way this condition can be distinguished with certainty from true endemic trachoma; smears and scrapings will yield the same information in both these conditions.

The treatment of inclusion SPK (TRIC virus) is the same as for hypoendemic trachoma, but the condition will settle in the end even without treatment, and without permanent damage.

OTHER FORMS OF CONJUNCTIVITIS

The conjunctiva looks a simple structure, but this is far from the truth. The entire surface of the eye and under surfaces of the lids are covered by it as a continuous mucous membrane, a membrane with a (sporadic) triple lamination, 2 to 5 cells thick depending on the site, and within which there are many goblet cells secreting mucus. The subjacent connective tissue is closely attached, that part closest to the overlying epithelium being profuscly infiltrated with lymphocytes; it is here inflammatory cells aggregate to form papillae and follicles when the conjunctiva is infected with micro-organisms, allergies, systemic viral diseases and exogenous irritants such as aerosol sprays. Adornment of the lid margins with a paste, especially in Asia, can cause an irritant conjunctivitis. The ingredients consist of soot and lead, or sometimes antimony, mixed with the fats of milk (ghee). In the deeper part of the subepithelial connective tissue layer lie the vessels and nerves supplying the conjunctiva. Increased mucous secretion, the presence of pus cells, increased vascularity and irregularities of the surface due to underlying papillary and follicular hypertrophy are the basic signs of any conjunctivitis. There is no photophobia until or unless the cornea is involved in the process, as it may. Only one segment of the bulbar conjunctiva may be affected as in phlyctenular conjunctivitis.

Acute bacterial conjunctivitis (purulent ophthalmia)

Bacterial infections vary in severity. *Pneumococcus,* The Koch Weeks bacillus and *Staphylococcus aureus* are the commonest organisms responsible, but any of the Gram-positive or negative bacteria may be involved. One or both eyes are affected, usually both. The organism should be identified under the microscope after staining (Ch. 7).

The attacks are often seasonal. Usually accompanied by mucopurulent or purulent discharge with matting of the eyelashes, the eyeball is either slightly or very congested (Plates 13, 14). Whatever the degree

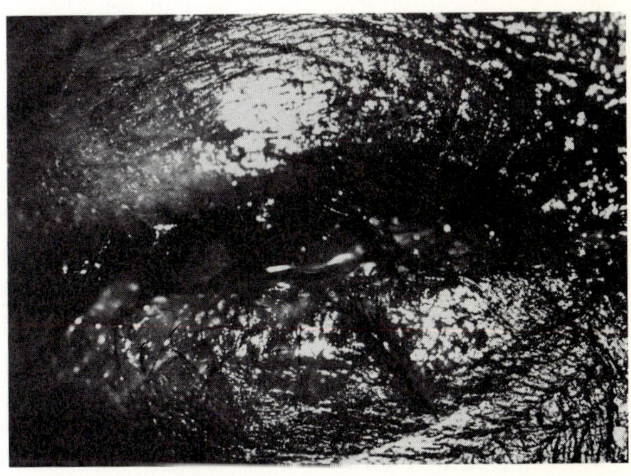

Plate 13 Secondary bacterial conjunctivitis in trachoma

of congestion, pain is not severe (a dull ache at the most); the cornea is clear, and the pupillary reactions are normal. Corneal foreign bodies, abrasions and ulcers should be sought by staining with Rose Bengal or fluorescein or both before making this diagnosis, especially if there is some pain. *If the pupil is smaller or larger in one eye than in the other, an anterior uveitis or an acute phase in a narrow angle glaucoma respectively may be the cause of the red eye, not conjunctivitis.*

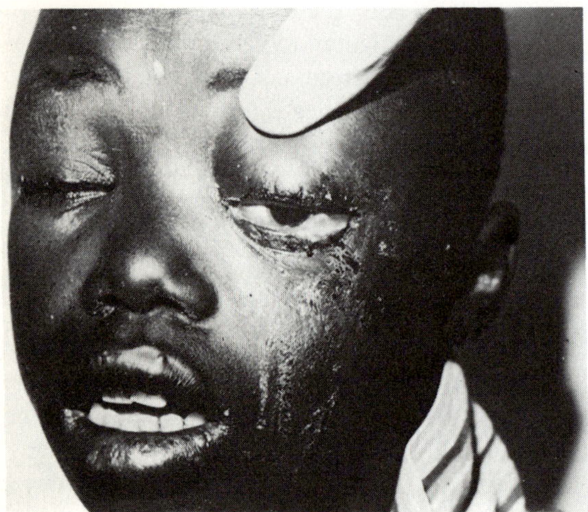

Plate 14 Purulent ophthalmia

Topical treatment thrice daily with a sulphonamide (such as sulphacetamide sodium 10 per cent) or a broad spectrum antibiotic (such as chloramphenicol 0.5 per cent) should bring an acute bacterial conjunctivitis under control in 3 to 4 days. Untreated, an acute bacterial conjunctivitis can reactivate a quiescent trachoma.

Acute viral conjunctivitis (non-TRIC)

The most common and serious kinds of viral conjunctivitis in the tropics have already been discussed under the headings of trachoma and the paratrachomas. Other viruses may be involved, however. In all viral infections the discharge is excessive, but watery or sticky, rarely purulent. Photophobia is common because generally the cornea is simultaneously involved. Non-TRIC viral infections reveal no inclusion bodies in pus cells and no bacteria in staining the secretion or conjunctival scrapings; they resist all treatment. These infections may last for a

month or longer before dying out. The two most characteristic are given below.

Epidemic punctate keratoconjunctivitis

The principal agent involved is adenovirus Type 8. It is an acute conjunctivitis with follicles on the palpebral conjunctiva, a densely congested, sometimes chemotic, bulbar conjunctiva, and many round, yellow, subepithelial corneal opacities, usually dispersed centrally, arising after a week or so. The preauricular lymph glands are swollen and tender. There is no fever, nor sore throat, as in Beal's conjunctivitis (syn. pharyngoconjunctival fever) which is otherwise identical. The condition slowly fades, but corneal opacities can last several months after the conjunctivitis has gone. The secretion is watery, but a mucofibrinous pseudomembrane usually can be found if sought in the lower fornix. A few examples of subconjunctival haemorrhage have been reported. Corneal involvement may reduce vision slightly for a week or longer at the peak of the disease (Fig. 3.9, 3.10 and Plate 15).

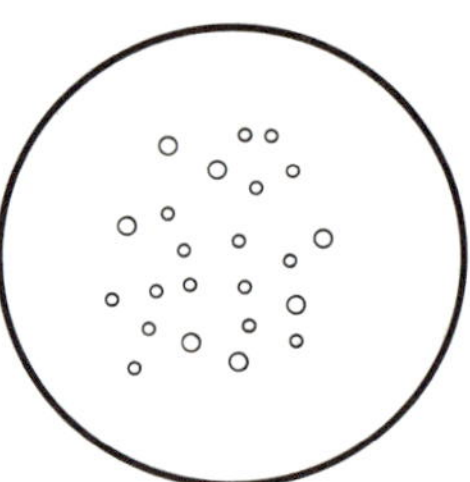

Fig. 3.9 Epidemic (punctate) keratoconjunctivitis. Average number and size of subepithelial opacities seen by direct illumination with the slit lamp

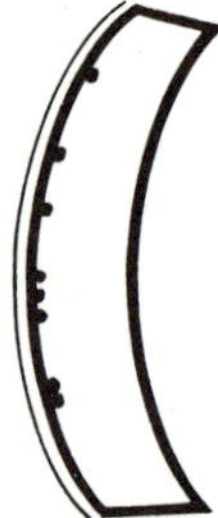

Fig. 3.10 Epidemic (punctate) keratoconjunctivitis. Subepithelial location of opacities seen in optical section of slit lamp

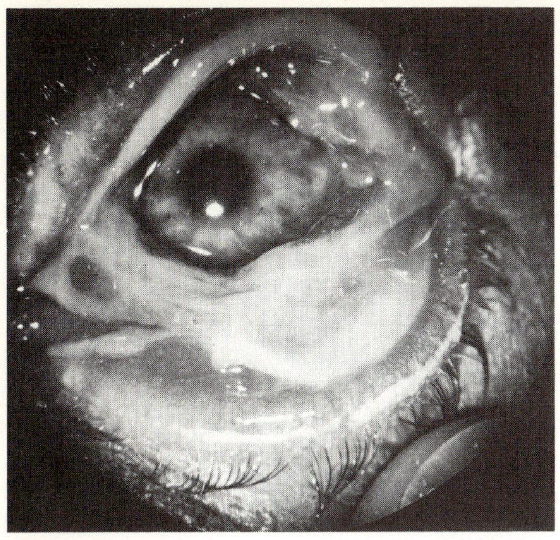

Plate 15 Pseudomembrane in epidemic (adenoviral) keratoconjunctivitis

Antibiotics and steroids are ineffective, but the former prevent secondary bacterial infection.

Epidemic haemorrhagic conjunctivitis

This condition was reported in vast numbers for the first time in Ghana by Chatterjee et al (1970). It has a quick onset with pain and swollen lids, lacrimation and a serous discharge, with enlargement of the preauricular lymph glands, as in the 'adenovirus 8' epidemic variety. There are follicles in the conjunctiva, and at that juncture the similarity ends. In only a handful of cases have subepithelial opacities been noted. Haemorrhages are characteristic, being present in all of the patients. They consist of a few pinpoint petechiae, or more rarely large blotches. Initially the haemorrhages are found in the conjunctiva covering the eyeball, near the fornix, increasing until the entire bulb is affected. Surprisingly, the conjunctivitis and the haemorrhages clear rapidly; it is claimed that 7 to 10 days is the limit. No adenovirus nor bacteria have been grown. It affects all ages and both sexes. There is no fever and no pharyngitis.

There is no specific treatment.

Chronic viral conjunctivitis

Many reports have emerged from India, where ocular health care is of a high standard, of conjunctival hyperaemia in young people, moving from one eye to the other. It responds to no known treatment, including antihistamines; bacteria and the classic adenoviruses have not to date been cultured. It is, nevertheless, most probably a viral infection of low virulence, although some believe it to be an allergic phenomenon.

Allergic conjunctivitis

There are three clinical entities that need to be recognised.

Phlyctenulosis (phlyctenular conjunctivitis)

The limbus at one point is the favoured site of a small, grey-white nodule (phlycten) (Plate 16), which is

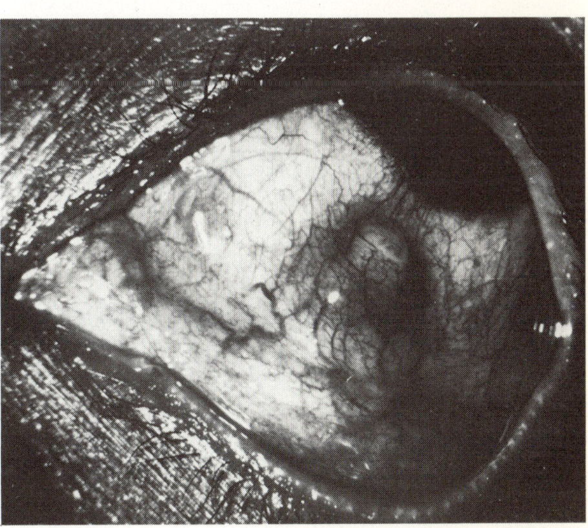

Plate 16 Bulbar phlycten. The patient also exhibited a tubercular choroiditis associated with miliary tuberculosis

always associated with a leash of blood vessels. The overlying epithelium frequently, though not invariably, breaks down; this necrotic area may spread into the cornea, followed by new vessels, giving rise to a phlyctenular corneal ulcer (also known as a 'fascicular' ulcer). It is most commonly seen in children, but young adults are also affected. It is generally unilateral. Usually, in the tropics, there is a generalised mild bulbar conjunctivitis associated with the phlycten.

Secondary infection can occur. The phlyctenular

ulcer may continue to spread across the cornea, followed by its proliferating blood vessels, or a second or third may arise elsewhere restricted to the limbus (Fig. 3.11). Rarely it leads to a perikeratitis.

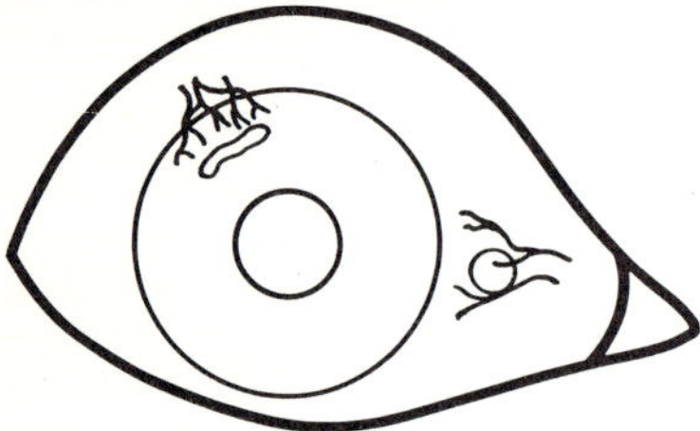

Fig. 3.11 Phlyctenulosis. A solitary phlycten on the bulbar conjunctiva nasally, and at the upper temporal limbus a marginal phlyctenular corneal ulcer

When the ulcer heals it leaves a 'half moon' scar at the limbus. This disease is often the result of sensitisation to a micro-organism, in particular to the human tubercle bacillus, frequently abdominal in India, but it is also found associated with gonorrhoea, leishmaniasis, trypanosomiasis, ascariasis and, rarely, with fungus infections. In all, it is a manifestation of delayed allergy.

In the tropics the general physical condition should be evaluated and attention especially directed towards tubercular disease of the lungs and abdomen, as well as to the nutrition of the patient.

The disease responds well to a topical mydriatic and steroid. An antibiotic to prevent secondary infection may be inserted at night.

Vernal (spring) catarrh

This condition is usually bilateral, and is more common in children than in adults. Its allergic nature is well established, but the allergen is not clear. It is not related to tubercle or malnutrition, as is so frequently phlyctenulosis. Over 60 per cent have other allergies. Clinically there are two forms of the disease: a palpebral and a limbal. The former is more common in areas where lightly pigmented eyes are found, the latter where darkly pigmented eyes are the rule, as in West Africa and Southern India.

Vernal catarrh of the palpebral conjunctiva. Large flat polyhedral granulations occur in the upper tarsal conjunctiva. They are packed together tightly (like cobblestones); they are pale-pink to grey in colour, and coated usually with a pale exudate. The conjunctiva of the lower lid has few or no cobblestones. The lesion, at first only irritable, because the cobblestones rub on the cornea, can cause abrasions; pain, marked photophobia and lacrimation develop later. The abrasions may advance to ulceration, and if infected, permanent scarring.

Vernal catarrh of the limbal conjunctiva. The lids are unaffected. The limbal conjunctiva is normally thicker than elsewhere, containing 10 or more layers of cells, including a high proportion of goblet cells. The entire ring of limbal epithelium (or part of it, less commonly) becomes swollen like a doughnut (known as limbal vernal catarrh). In the pigmented eye it is densely black. Being irritable, rubbing may produce corneal ulceration. It does not spread onto the cornea more than a few mm.

Both limbal and palpebral varieties of vernal catarrh respond well to topical steroids, but applications may have to be prolonged; small doses of systemic steroid for short periods are even more effective, and there is little difference in the overall cost.

NUTRITIONAL XEROPHTHALMIA

Vitamin A deficiency

Of all blinding diseases in developing countries, xerophthalmia and cataract are the most universal. Xerophthalmia is the more tragic, because it is avoidable, being due to a deficiency of vitamin A.

Vitamin A deficiency may affect many parts of the body and can be a contributory cause of death. In man, particularly in children, the most striking features consist of ocular changes which affect the health of the external ocular membranes, the corneal stroma and the retina, reducing the sensitivity of the latter to light, so that vision in the dark becomes poor to the point of night blindness. As the external ocular lesions are not only the most striking, but the most common, and can progress to blindness without death occurring, xerophthalmia may be considered an ocular entity. Nevertheless, it cannot often be divorced from systemic changes, so in the back of the clinician's mind, the vitamin A status of the individual, and those factors affecting that status which cause it to become poor or marginal or acceptable, must always be present.

Because vitamin A is largely stored in the liver, deficiency can be hastened as a result of defective storage (as in hepatic cirrhosis, frequently postinfective), or again, where there is difficulty in absorbing it (or its pro-vitamin) from the intestine (as in sprue, gastroenteritis and kwashiorkor), or where there is excessive usage of/demand for vitamin A (as in fevers such as measles, malaria or pneumonia).

It is not so very long ago that a prerequisite before diagnosing xerophthalmia in any region was the collection of *quantitative dietary intake* data. That some ocular cases occurred did not then matter, provided the intake was found to be adequate.

The author in 1953/54 in North Nigeria, when reporting the presence of clinical cases of xerophthalmia, and biochemical determinations (8) which yielded low blood values, was told *dietary intake data* refuted his findings, and that there was no vitamin A deficiency problem. This is now known to have been incorrect in the very area in which the work was carried out, but it took many years to establish the realities.

Probability surveys based on the clinical presence of xerophthalmia and biochemical determinations where possible are now accepted as the real criteria. 'Only then can dietary investigations aimed at providing quantitative data be usefully conducted as part of an intensive follow-up investigation as one of several bases for choosing an appropriate intervention program' (IVACG Report, 1976). This statement places dietary surveys in their true perspective.

It must be clear by now that where the dietary intake of pro-vitamin beta-carotene and vitamin A in a district is apparently adequate, when dealing with the individual with malabsorption from the intestine, perhaps faced with an extra demand for vitamin A by reason of some infection, the balance can become easily tilted from an 'acceptable' to a 'marginal' or 'poor' level of vitamin A. This is particularly pertinent in the case of a weanling or growing child.

Protein malnutrition

It is important to distinguish between protein energy malnutrition (PEM) and protein deficiency. These are two opposite ends of a spectrum, *often confused by reason of intermediate syndromes.*

Nutritional marasmus

This is the commonest and most dramatic form of PEM. In this condition there is a shortage of protein with an associated caloric deficiency. It is characterised by severe wasting away of fat and muscle. The classic picture is of a markedly underweight child, reduced to skin and bone, with a big head, staring, apathetic eyes and a wizened old face. There is in a true nutritional marasmus an *absence* of hair changes, 'flaky-paint' dermatosis, dyspigmentation, hepatomegaly and oedema, the latter all being striking findings when present in kwashiorkor (see below). Cases are seen which are intermediate (marasmic kwashiorkor) where there is wasting and oedema and some of the signs of kwashiorkor just given. Any form may be complicated or initiated by chronic gastroenteritis or other infections (such as tuberculosis).

Kwashiorkor

This condition is due to protein deficiency alone with caloric *sufficiency* from carbohydrate foods. Constant findings include growth retardation and oedema, commencing in the feet and lower legs, then involving the hands, thighs, sacrum, back, arms and face. The third constant finding is a decrease in muscle and an increase in body fat, and the fourth is apathy. The plasma proteins are always low, especially serum albumin.

Variable findings in kwashiorkor include hair changes (Plate 17): lightening or change of colour—

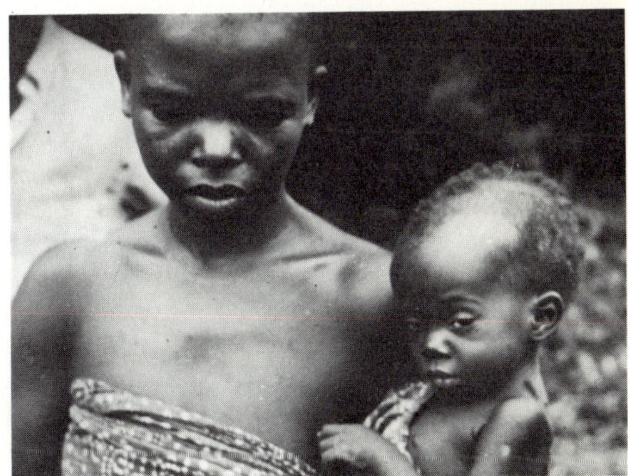

Plate 17 African child with kwashiorkor. Note hair changes

reddish brown is common in the dark-haired—sparseness, increased softness and loss of curliness in hair, and hair that is easily pulled out (pelo facilmente desprendibile). In addition to these hair changes, 'flaky-paint' dermatosis, loose stools due to malabsorption, hepatomegaly and anaemia may occur. Kwashiorkor may be distinguished from nephrosis with oedema, as in the latter the urine is loaded with protein, whereas in kwashiorkor it is never more than slight.

Vitamin A deficiency and protein energy malnutrition frequently co-exist and in the child there may in addition be a defective immunological defence mechanism and multiple infections. It is in such children that xerosis (dryness of the external eye) develops, and can advance to keratomalacia (necrosis of the cornea). These changes, and any intermediate ones, come under the heading of nutritional xerophthalmia.

Ocular features

The changes just described in the last paragraph above do not inevitably follow one another. Moreover, they may be so slight that they are overlooked, which makes it all the more important to consider the general health of a patient under observation.

Basic changes

Xerosis is a non-specific term used in ophthalmology to describe a pathological change of the cornea or conjunctiva, or both, which follows hyperkeratosis (keratinisation) of the surface epithelium of the eyeball. It is found in scars from any cause, in degenerations associated with dystrophic conditions, in the more advanced stages of an inflammatory process, in exposure keratitis, and so on. That is why it is more precise to use the term 'nutritional' when discussing a xerosis caused by a nutritional defect. It is the epithelium which is primarily affected. In chapter 2 of this book, the role of mucus in maintaining the health of the corneal and conjunctival epithelium is described, but in no instance, even in long untreated cases, has a keratoconjunctivitis sicca been known to advance to xerosis in the absence of vitamin A deficiency. When mucus is abnormal, as it is in sicca lesions, multiple minute erosions arise, never hyperkeratosis; so although the mucus sec-

reted by the conjunctival epithelial goblet cells may be deficient, in vit. A deficiency it is not abnormal in consistency, and is unlikely to play more than a secondary role in the production of the fully developed lesion known as nutritional xerosis. To support this view, the skin lesion most characteristic of vitamin A deficiency takes the form of a hyperkeratosis; here the skin is dry, atrophic and scaly and the hair follicles are enlarged. The association between xerophthalmia and hyperkeratosis of the skin in vitamin A deficiency has been reported by many workers for a long time and supplies a ready explanation of the changes which occur in the eye.

Nutritional xerosis

These changes are restricted to the bulbar conjunctiva in the first instance, and to the temporal side. It is common in the tropics up to the age of 10. In consequence of the thickening of the conjunctival epithelium, the papilliform surface is smoothed out and the tears are unable to adhere to the affected part by surface tension despite the presence of mucus of more or less normal consistency; the affected area in consequence looks dry, is dry, loses its lustre, loses its transparency, loses its tone, wrinkles concentric to the limbus, and becomes in the end pigmented. The longer untreated the patient is the larger will the area become and the grosser the changes just described. It is possible that the localised lesions, known as Bitot's spots (Plate 18), reflect a milder form of nutritional xerosis of the conjunctiva of this type, restricted to the most exposed area of the bulb. Alternatively, the spots may represent an aborted nutritional xerosis. Whatever their origin, Bitot's spots are not necessarily associated with low serum vitamin A or with nutritional xerosis, nor with any other evidence of vitamin A deficiency, and they do not as a rule respond to vitamin A therapy. What is certain is that Bitot's spots only occur in situations where malnutrition exists. Although the keratinised areas of the eyeball are slightly coated with mucus, other debris when present, whatever its nature, also becomes attached. The silvery white, conglomerate secretion provided by bacterial saprophytes such as *Corynebacterium xerosis* or *Moraxella lacunata* not infrequently adheres to a Bitot's spot, which becomes 'pearly' in appearance; if the nutritional xerosis is more widespread, scattered linear deposits of this same secretion con-

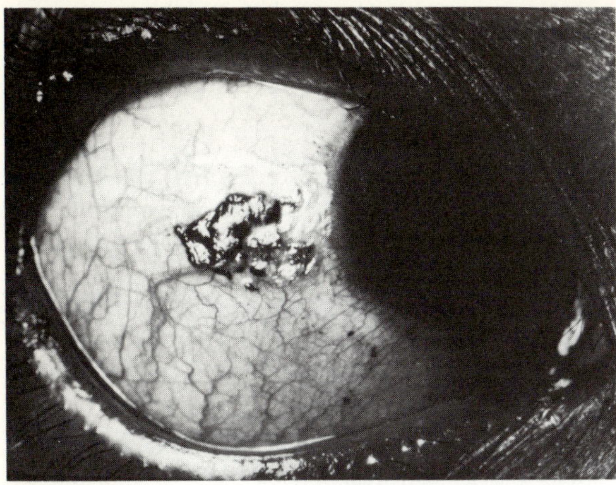

Plate 18 Lamp black adherent to localised bulbar hyperkeratosis (Bitot's spot)

centric with the limbus occur; in an infected red eye some of the mucopurulent secretion may attach itself to the roughened area of bulbar epithelium, and this has been called a 'mucoid' spot (Rodger, 1963).

If nutritional xerosis persists and is untreated, it will increasingly involve the bulbar conjunctiva, affecting the lower fornix and the cornea (Plate 19).

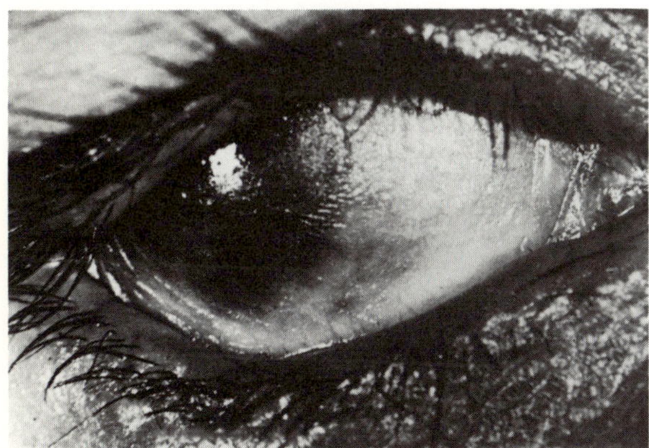

Plate 19 Nutritional xerosis of conjunctiva and part of cornea

The latter becomes *patchily* dry, then wholly dry. In the optical section of the slit lamp, a thickening of the corneal epithelium is apparent, and infiltration of the anterior stroma arises. Later the entire cornea loses its lustre. With Rose Bengal stain there are fewer erosions in the anterior segment of the eye than one would expect in these circumstances, but there is still a considerable number. The loss of translucency of

the cornea described above advances until it becomes densely opaque, especially at the apex, which is the thinnest sector. It is at the apex that the hyperkeratinised epithelium first exhibits cracks or facets, and it is the corneal apex on healing which invariably exhibits a permanent scar (leucoma).

Keratomalacia

Where malnutrition is rife, as in parts of Central and South America, Africa and Asia, and exacerbated in the weanling by measles, malaria or pneumonia, one finds kwashiorkor and nutritional marasmus. It is in such patients one finds classic keratomalacia (Plates 20 and 21). However, these associations, and

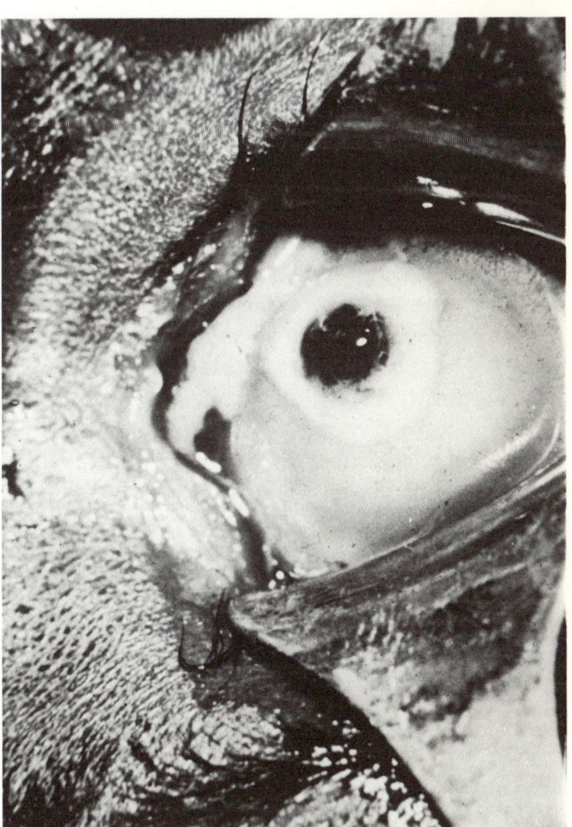

Plate 20 Acute keratomalacia

the co-existence of HSV ulcers (sometimes blamed as the basic cause of keratomalacia) are not found in all cases, any more than the belief that keratomalacia necessarily follows nutritional xerosis. In short, this

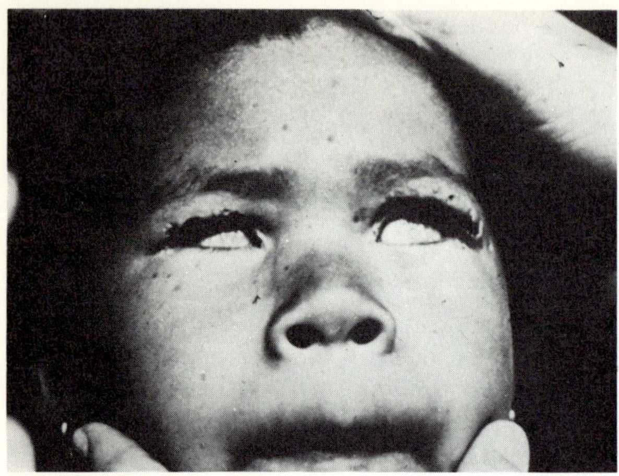

Plate 21 Healed blinding keratomalacia

condition is not fully understood. The epidemiological evidence is against HSV being anything other than a rare cause. Recent work has strengthened the view that it has quite a different pathogenesis from nutritional xerosis and ties it in with an absence of an anticollagenase factor in the cornea or in the blood. Nevertheless, it does happen that nutritional xerosis of the cornea can advance to ulceration, the cornea can perforate and the final picture can resemble keratomalacia. The striking feature of keratomalacia, reported by many workers, is that initially it is a quiet condition with very little reaction and no ulceration. Even after the cornea has spontaneously ruptured, severe secondary infection may never occur. With so many possible adverse features involved, it is not surprising the clinical picture has been so variously described in different regions.

Localised depressions indicative of thinning are the first sign that keratomalacia may be pending. These need not commence at the corneal apex, but anywhere on the cornea. Suddenly such a facet perforates or becomes so thin that, as only Descement's membrane remains, the aqueous under pressure is able to push a knuckle of iris outwards, still covered by the membrane (syn. Descemetocele). Blood vessels enter the cornea at the site of these areas of corneal necrosis, but even then there may be no acute inflammatory reaction. The process continues until the entire cornea has broken up and disappeared. The front of the eye now consists of uvea, some corneal collagen and Descemet's membrane, the whole bound together by exudate, with the lens

and vitreous pressing forward against this precarious barrier from behind.

Nutritional myocephalon

This term, literally 'the head of a fly', was used by Rodger & Sinclair (1969) to describe a spontaneous small round black iris prolapse, seen in the corneas of children in poor areas. It is in fact an old term dating back to the 19th century. Blumenthal (1950) called it malnutritional keratitis, a term of little merit, but the credit of noting it first is his. The myocephalon is found in underweight children, and the serum vitamin A blood levels are generally rather low. It is a painless, symptomless, small, clean iris prolapse, sometimes covered by Descemet's, 2 to 3 mm in diameter, occurring generally close to the limbus, usually in the lower half of the cornea, usually single but not always, and invariably without any local reaction whatsoever. The lesion appears to heal spontaneously, especially if the child's state of nutrition is moderately good.

The treatment of this interesting condition is symptomatic. It can be lightly touched with phenol.

Night blindness

The International Vitamin A Consultative Group (IVACG) has classified night blindness as a secondary sign (symptom?) of xerophthalmia, along with a xerophthalmia fundus, postxerotic corneal scars and Bitot's spots 'when unaccompanied by nutritional xerosis'. Bitot's spots and corneal scars (leucomata) have already been discussed, and the so-called xerophthalmia fundus is extremely rare. It is better known as Lauber's or Uyemara's syndrome.* The probability of a misdiagnosis exists unless the examiner is most experienced or a measurable night blindness is found to co-exist. A miniature dark adaptometer has been designed for use in the field (Rodger, 1976). This instrument is used to measure the minimal light theshold and visual acuity in a dark adapted eye, and is ideal for field work and the small clinic (see Ch. 1) Early studies in Panama, Papua New Guinea and Sulawesi, involving 500 children over the age of 7, confirm previous findings that

*The verbal description IVACG gives of the retinal changes corresponds very closely to a common variety of hyaline degeneration of the retina, and is not very convincing.

night blindness in the absence of xerosis is common in the tropics. This instrument enables the practitioner to measure the potential threat of vitamin A deficiency by assessing its prevalence in a community. It is quick and easy to use.

Treatment

Two maxims should be considered before commencing treatment of nutritional xerophthalmia: (1) if nutritional xerosis of the cornea is treated early, the condition can be reversed and *sight* saved; (2) if keratomalacia can be treated early, the condition can be arrested, some sight salvaged and *life* saved.

It should be noted that spontaneous cures arise in both types of disorder, nutritional xerosis and keratomalacia, especially in a peasant farming community with pre-harvest starvation, where new supplies of essential foodstuffs may become available before xerophthalmia has advanced too far. Recovery often depends on whether the mother takes the trouble to feed and nurse her child. Other nutritional deficiencies, such as ariboflavinosis (maceration of the nostrils and edges of the mouth) must be looked for and treated.

Use of vitamin A preparations

The following procedure is recommended for both nutritional xerosis and keratomalacia.

Retinyl palmitate is a preferred active form of vitamin A in water-miscible form for intramuscular injection. Vitamin A acetate is used orally. In keratomalacia, red palm oil of high carotene content has been found useless, presumably because it is not absorbed or converted in the affected intestine.

Regimen:

1st Day   100 000 IU retinyl palmitate intramuscularly
2nd Day   100 000 IU vitamin A acetate orally
3rd Day   50 000 IU vitamin A acetate orally daily
to
7th Day

Toxic effects (headache, pruritus and nausea) are unlikely with this dosage, which it is known can be tolerated for much longer. Thereafter a diet as rich in vitamin A as possible should be given.

Use of protein and carbohydrate

In keratomalacia a high protein diet is required, milk in children being the basis. Glucose is added to the milk in the early stages of treatment, as hypoglycaemia is invariably present. An intake of 100 cal/kg should be the aim. At the start 2g of potassium is needed daily. Although there is retention of sodium, the level falls when treatment is underway, and additional sodium chloride (1 to 2g daily) is soon needed. In severe dehydrated cases a gastric or i.v. infusion may be necessary. Topical and/or systemic antibiotic therapy may be required for any co-existing infections of eye or body (such as the lungs, or the bowels), and if possible should be given routinely. Intramuscular iron will cure anaemia, and it is advisable also to treat routinely for malaria. It is the association of infections such as these which leads to the high mortality rate and the high incidence of blindness in such patients, hence the importance of using every possible aid.

Prevention

Prevention of nutritional xerophthalmia in young children may be attempted by encouraging mothers to breast-feed and to eat beta-carotene contained in foods such as pawpaw, string beans (including the leaves) and palm oil during pregnancy and lactation. Breast-feeding up to two years or more is customary in developing countries, and almost universally successful among tropical peasant mothers. Its value is shown by the usual excellent rate of growth during the first 6 months of life (or longer), and the absence generally of PEM and vitamin A deficiency during this period. The protein and vitamin A content of breast milk, even from poorly fed mothers, is now well recognised to be normal even in late lactation. Thus prolonged lactation in the poorer of the developing countries is a most valuable asset to offset PEM, and one to be preserved and, if possible, augmented by introducing after 6 months or a year easily digestible foods, especially vegetable and animal proteins, thereby avoiding the disastrous combination of vitamin A and protein deficiencies. To ensure this occurs requires health education at the village level.

Leaf protein (LP) made by a simple extraction of fresh green leaves, followed by heat precipitation of the protein, is now known to be a rich source of the pro-vitamin beta-carotene. Pirie (1978) has established LP as an acceptable source of protein, especially useful in areas where milk is scarce, despite initial scepticism, and even hostility, at his proposals. Peasant farmers should be encouraged to grow more leaves. The darker the leaf, the redder the fruit, and the deeper the yellow colour of a root crop, the more pro-vitamin beta-carotene is likely to be present for manufacture and consumption.

ONCHOCERCIASIS (river blindness)

Natural history

River blindness is found in Africa approximately between 15°N and 15°S as well as in Guatemala, Venezuela, Mexico and Columbia (slightly). There are also small foci in North Sudan and the Yemen.

For the benefit of those unfamiliar with the disease, we must consider three living things: man, the fly which infects him, and the worm which multiplies in his body. The fly breeds in running water (hence the term river blindness) and belongs to a species of the genus *Simulium*. Shortly after the fly feeds on man, the offspring of the adult worms (called *microfilariae)* can be detected in the fly's stomach with the blood meal; they vary in size from 285 to 360 μm. Within about 24 hours they wander from the stomach into the fly's muscles, usually those of the thorax. Here they settle down and undergo changes in shape, and after about a week they have changed into the longer and thinner 'infective larvae' which migrate to the salivary glands of the fly. When the fly next has a blood meal it deposits these 'infective larvae' on the skin of another human being, and the larvae penetrate through the bite. They then grow gradually into adult worms; but their offspring, the microfilariae, cannot grow into adults until they in turn pass through a fly.

The worm which is the cause of all the trouble belongs to a group known as filarial worms, and is called *Onchocerca* (literally 'hook tail'). As its body has a spiral groove, it is specifically designated as *Onchocerca volvulus* in Africa, *O. caecutiens* in Central and South America. The latter has certain physiological differences (especially its mf.) and may be a distinct species. The natural history of *O. caecutiens* in man differs somewhat from *O. volvulus*, although it is believed to have come from Africa in the bodies of slaves.

In the early stages the adult worms lie free, but later they live in tumours (called nodules or onchocercomas) in the subcutaneous tissues or deeper planes of the body (in particular in the head in America). The size of the nodules varies widely as does their number; over 20 may be counted. The fibrous tissue which encapsules the male and female *Onchocerca* is a reaction of the body to the worms. The worms are white opalescent nematodes, tapering at both ends, the tail of the female being curved like a hook. Females attain a length of 30 to 50 cm and a transverse diameter of 270 to 400 μm; the males are much smaller, 1.9 to 4.2 cm, with diameters of 130 to 210 μm. Thus free 'worms' can be found of any length between 285 μm and 50 cm. If only female worms are present in the nodule, no young are produced and the infection dies out in that site. Usually there are many male and female worms present, coiled round each other. They are believed to live for at least 15 years. The young, the microfilariae, are produced in tremendous numbers, migrating easily through the nodule into the skin. Counts of more than 2000 mf./10 mg of skin are not uncommon; they probably live for 6 months (Crewe and Wéry, 1977). Their natural habitat is extravascular; they are only rarely found in the bloodstream, a fact more commonly reported in recent years. As the number of adults in the host increases so does the number of the microfilariae which spread further afield under the skin; when they reach the eyelids they pass readily under the conjunctiva; from there, passage into the orbit or into the eye is a simple matter. The larvae penetrate the inner eye (and no doubt elsewhere) most easily by passing down the loose adventitial sheaths of the perforating vessels. This occurs not only in the anterior ocular segment, but not surprisingly also in the posterior. In this way the microfilariae have access to all ocular structures and tissues. The range of penetration into other structures of the body organs seems unlimited, and is only now becoming apparent (Rodger, 1959).

The popular name for the fly vector is 'the black fly'. The genus Simulium is widespread. The species responsible for transmitting onchocerciasis in West Africa down to and including Angola is *S. damnosum* Theobald; in East Africa, down to Eastern Zaire, another species, *S. neavei* Roubaud, also acts as a vector. Other species of *Simulium* are involved in Central America and Mexico (*S. ochraceum* and *S. metallicum*). The distribution of river blindness does not necessarily correspond to that of onchocerciasis of the skin, nor does that of cutaneous onchocerciasis to that of the vector. This is because, in the first instance, the disease may be so minor that it does not affect the eye: and in the second, because in some regions the fly does not bite man, or because the climatic conditions reduce the life span of the insect to such an extent that it bites man only once during its lifetime, and is thus incapable of transmitting *infective* larvae.

The black flies are somewhat less than one-quarter the size of the house fly. Their eggs are laid beneath flowing water preferentially where the streams and rivers are swift. This factor is not infrequently absent in large slower-flowing rivers. The eggs are usually deposited on substrates such as rocks or vegetation under water. Those of *S. neavei* are also laid on river crabs. Eggs develop into larvae and then pupae, finally to emerge from the river as adult flies, which rest and breed on the banks. It is the pregnant female which preys on riverine man and keeps ever increasing the huge human reservoir of onchocerciasis, which is thought to consist of at least 20 million people in Africa and 5 million in Central and South America. The danger of the disease spreading to other countries is a very real one, if one thinks in terms of centuries.

Development of the lesions

Wherever *mf. volvulus* die, the bodies disintegrate and act as a toxin, causing direct damage to adjacent cells. As there may be many dead or dying mf. in any single small area, the damage can be severe, not only to the structures of the eye, but to the dermal subepithelium of the skin and its capillaries. The capillary endothelium swells until the small vessels close and atrophy; the resultant anoxia accentuates the tissue necrosis, initially caused by the toxins emanating from mf. dissolution. Thick, atrophic, non-elastic skin (pacchydermia) with depigmentation and excoriation due to scratching results, particularly on the legs. Uneven pigmentation and papular eruptions of the skin are early changes well seen over the buttocks. Enlarged lymph nodes around the groin occur. When multiple they stretch the skin to produce a 'hanging groin'; interference with the lymphatic flow can lead to elephantiasis. In the upper lids pseudo-ptosis ('bung' eye) in advanced cases may be seen; oedema is the initial cause followed by the development of myxomatous tissue. Strangely enough, there is not a very close relationship between the number of mf. in the cornea as an isolated early phenomenon—it is known as a punctate keratitis (PK) because the mf. are dispersed—and the number of mf. in the skin. Where counts of up to 20 mf. in the cornea are concerned, the number present is apparently dictated by chance. In the case of counts over 20, one would have thought that chance was less likely to influence the number present, and a significant relationship might be expected with skin counts; this has not been demonstrated either. Indeed the opposite has been sometimes found. Thus, as far as the punctate keratitis of onchoceriasis is concerned, the number of mf. present seems to be dictated entirely by chance above a certain density of skin infection.

Microfilariae appear in the cornea earlier than in the anterior chamber, and can be seen in both in children. Contrary to what one finds in the cornea, there *is* a close relationship between the number of mf. in the anterior chamber and the skin infectivity. The highest proportion of eyes with mf. in the anterior chamber occurs in the 30 to 40 age group, although a not inconsiderable number of the eyes of children at puberty are also invaded. When present in the young the numbers are higher than in most adults, 50 or more mf. having been counted within the anterior chamber. Sclerosing keratitis is, as in the case of mf. in the anterior chamber, associated with higher microfilarial skin counts than in onchocercal patients with healthy eyes, irrespective of the age of the patients.

The uveal changes are somewhat different, especially the severe, for they (like PK patients) do not have a close relationship with skin mf. density. There is increasing evidence that within hyperendemic areas a group exists among those infected which is more susceptible to uveal lesions than the remainder of the population, for the level of onchocerca antibody has been found to be higher in those with uveal lesions than in those without. Rodger & Maertens (1977) found a percentage of those with affected uveas under 40 years of age had relatively lower levels of skin infection than those with healthy eyes. Over 40 years of age there is little difference. This strengthens the argument that there is a group more susceptible to developing uveal lesions than the average, and explains why in a population where everybody appears to be heavily infected only a small proportion has seriously impaired vision of one or both eyes.

The posterior degenerative lesion of onchocerciasis has an obscure origin, which cannot be associated with any of the factors mentioned above. Microfilariae have been found rarely in the optic nerve and retina, frequently in the choroid, so the severity of this lesion may vary with the number and situation of dead mf. in these structures. Some form of 'larva migrans' has been suggested recently as a cause, present as two, perhaps three, small, immature adults (Rodger & Maertens, 1977). The changes found in the optic nerve will be discussed in the section entitled 'The problem of optic atrophy'.

Ocular features

As only a small percentage of biting black flies contain infective stage larvae, and as a generality they prefer to bite legs in Africa and heads in Central America, infection is usually avoided by those who merely travel through endemic areas, or who work there for only a short time, or who wear hats and long trousers. The number of blind in the community, as has been mentioned above, varies considerably from under 1 per cent to 20 per cent. A prevalence rate of 10 per cent or over may be considered high. Examination of those between 30 and 40 years of age most quickly indicates the severity of river blindness in a town, for within the third decade of life the disease either remains as it is, or dies out (leaving little or no damage to the eyes), or advances rapidly in a proportion of men and women of this decade to produce severe loss of sight.

Before 30 years of age, ocular involvement is common, but is usually of moderate severity, if we exclude the posterior degenerative lesion, which can be severe at all ages. Early changes are entirely those of invasion of the anterior segment of the eye by many mf. volvulus, (PK and mf. in anterior chamber) and seldom cause permanent damage. After the third decade, however, the lesions become more widespread, more serious and more diverse, depending partly upon repeated invasion and death, and

partly upon hypersensitivity to the toxins.

Punctate keratitis and larvae in the anterior chamber

The most common early distribution is one of erratic dispersal of mf. over the entire cornea. When alive and moving, *mf. volvulus* are nearly impossible to see in the cornea unless close to the epithelium. The static appearance of linear and fluffy opacities up to 0.5 mm in length at all levels in the stroma results from the presence of dead larvae. If subepithelial, these may be called a superficial punctate keratitis; an interstitial keratitis occurs when inflammatory cells surround dispersed groups of dead mf. volvulus in the stroma (Buck, 1974).

Biomicroscopically, the larvae in the anterior chamber are best seen in the line of the beam as minute, wriggling objects in the aqueous, their colour depending on the brightness of the incident light. Sometimes patients complain of entopic phenomena due to their lashing movements; usually around 50 mf. are present when such a complaint is received. Quite commonly mf. are seen with their heads pressed against the posterior corneal surface, especially low down, or against the anterior lens capsule. They may remain there for a few seconds, writhing violently as if stuck, and then are gone into the 'pool' of aqueous. Mf. have been noted in the retrolental space of Berger, and a few in the vitreous.

Nummular opacities are not uncommon in African eyes, but also exist in areas where there is no onchocerciasis; they may be viral or due to trauma and need not be discussed further.

Sclerosing keratitis

The classical corneal change in onchocerciasis is sclerosing keratitis. The keratitis commences at 3 or 9 o'clock, from where 'tongues' of *pannus onchocercosus* invade the cornea; in the end they may meet at the centre. Another common appearance is as an 'apron' of pannus around the lower half of the cornea; this lesion also advances towards the pupillary area (Plate 22). Several tongues of pannus can appear at the same time in the lower half of the cornea, all becoming confluent in the end. When the condition is allowed to advance unchecked, the end-result is total involvement of the cornea; such a pannus advances

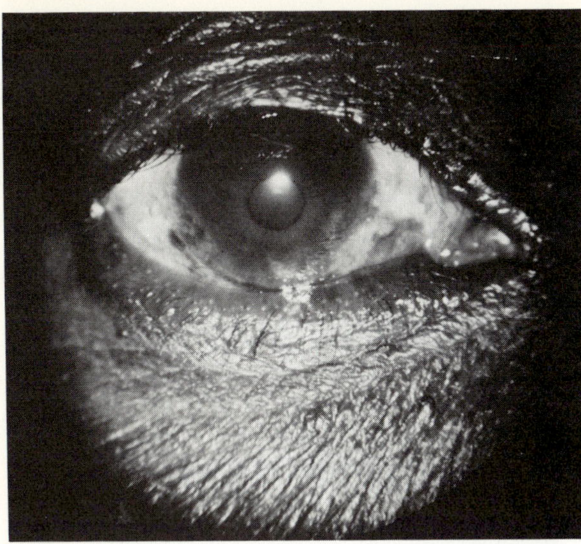

Plate 22 Onchocercal sclerosing keratitis (apron in lower cornea)

until all that is left is a clear area (of cornea) at 12 o'clock (Figs 3.12 and 3.13).

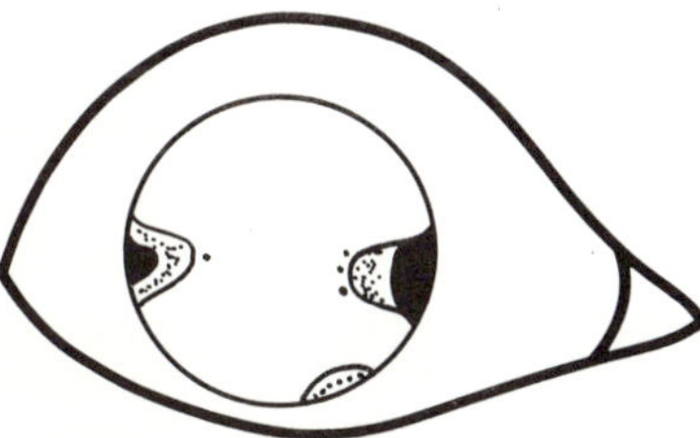

Fig. 3.12 Onchocercal sclerosing keratitis developing from 'tongues' at 3 and 9 o'clock, with a smaller lesion at 5 o'clock. The three zones are shown in the diagram: grey, white and pigmented

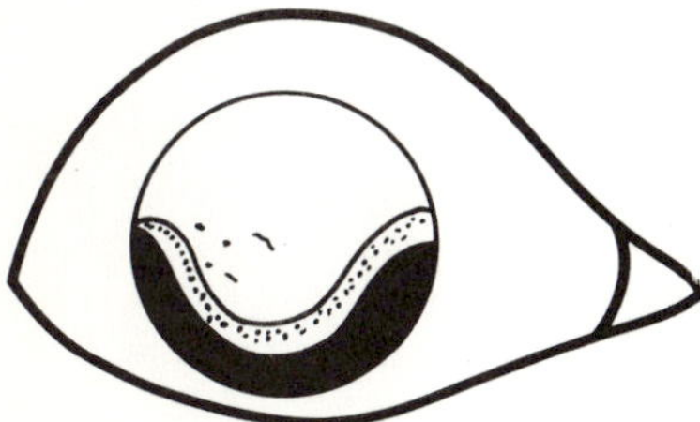

Fig. 3.13 The 'tongues' have now joined to form an apron of corneal opacification, classically always in the lower half of the cornea

The external appearance of the *pannus onchocerco-sus* is fairly characteristic: it lies at first between the epithelium and Bowman's membrane, as would a *pannus degenerativus*, but differs from the latter in being vascularised. Subsequently, it may break through Bowman's membrane, or appear well below it. It is often associated (when the cornea is invaded by mf. in force) with interstitial areas of fibrosis. The pannus consists of three zones: an advancing 'snow-storm' zone of separate grey dots, a middle, white zone, where the individual opacifications (infiltrates) are densely packed, and a basal pigmented zone. In the end, the epithelial surface above the pannus may become entirely pigmented, although it can be seen under high magnification to fade off towards the upper pole of the cornea. Corneal neovascularisation is essentially restricted to the pannus, although in late cases, as indicated, new, large blood vessels may enter the stroma. At all stages in this condition, one finds evidence of corneal degenerations, such as band-shaped keratopathy. The keratitis is quite frequently associated with an anterior uveitis.

Anterior uveitis

About 60 per cent of all defective sight resulting from onchocerciasis arises from anterior uveal inflammation and its complications. The condition is generally seen as an insidious, low-grade, nongranulomatous infection, or even when it has been severe, in a quiescent state; there seems little doubt that occasional short-lived bursts of acute or subacute uveal

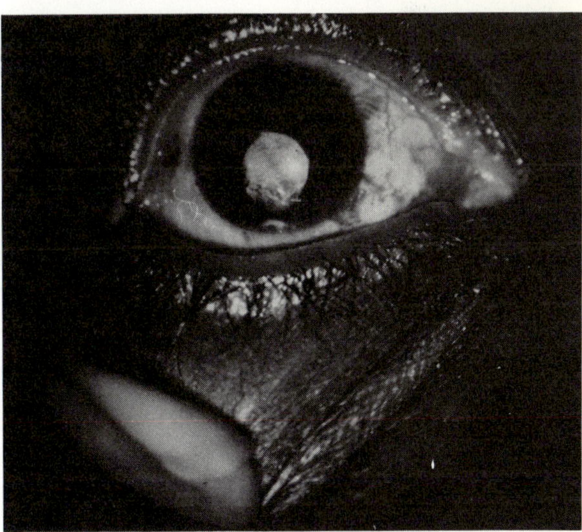

Plate 23 Onchocercal exudate concealing complicated cataract and spilling into anterior chamber

activity occur, as they have been witnessed in field surveys.

The iris changes are noticeable at the pupillary margin. There is loss of pigment from the frill, exudation in front of, across or behind the pupil, formation of posterior adhesions usually associated with entropion (inturning) of the pupil and keratic precipitates. The latter are pigmented and small, rarely lardaceous (mutton fat). A gelatinous exudate (Plate 23) occasionally spills over into the anterior chamber at 6 o'clock, dragging the pupil margin down and outwards (hence the term ectropion of the pupillary margin); an oval or pear-shaped pupil may result. The exudate, when it has become organised, becomes grey or white in colour. Not uncommonly, circles or parts of cirlces, blue-white in colour, run round the pupillary margin, or even cover the entire pupil. This appearance has been called 'flocculation' for convenience (Plate 24). In an endemic area, it is a

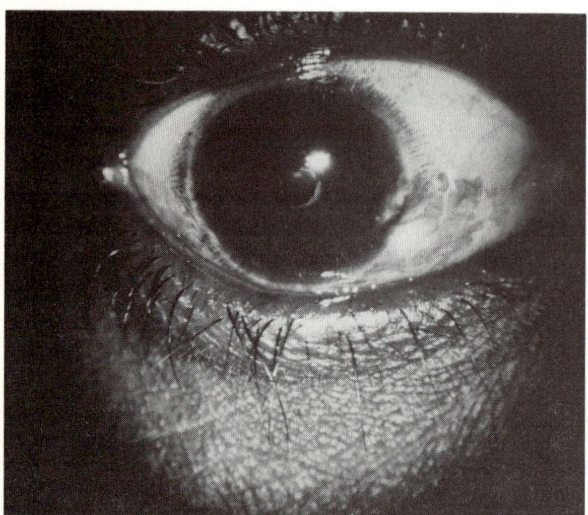

Plate 24 Flocculation around pupillary margin in onchocercal anterior uveitis

specific sign. In severe anterior uveitis, occlusion of the pupil, or seclusion, with secondary glaucoma is not uncommon; the iris crypts may be filled in, giving a brown flat iris with the appearance of velvet. Complicated cataracts may be seen to have arisen and the choroid may also be affected.

Posterior segmental lesions

The changes in the choroid are frequently concealed by inflammatory membranes resulting from anterior uveitis, membranes either covering the front of the lens, or where the ciliary processes have been involved covering the posterior surface of the lens (cyclitic membrane), thereby concealing the posterior segmental changes. Where a complicated cataract exists, it is also impossible to see these changes. Where invasion of the entire uvea is gross, and this has been frequently shown histopathologically, a disseminated chorioretinitis occurs; there may be only a single focus, but generally there are several; they may be circumscribed, diffuse, central, paracentral or peripheral, but in all cases there is the same underlying pathology, namely focal necrosis, oedema, cell infiltration and fragmented larvae, associated with chorioretinal scarring and fusion and varying degrees of vascular closure of the exposed underlying choroidal vessels.

Optic atrophy is a common cause of blindness in onchocerciasis and is discussed fully in the section entitled 'The problem of optic atrophy' in Chapter 4.

The classic change in onchocerciasis involving the posterior segment of the eye is often called *the Hissette-Ridley fundus* (Plate 25). Paradoxically, the histopathology is not in accord with that just recounted, unless one presupposes that it follows the

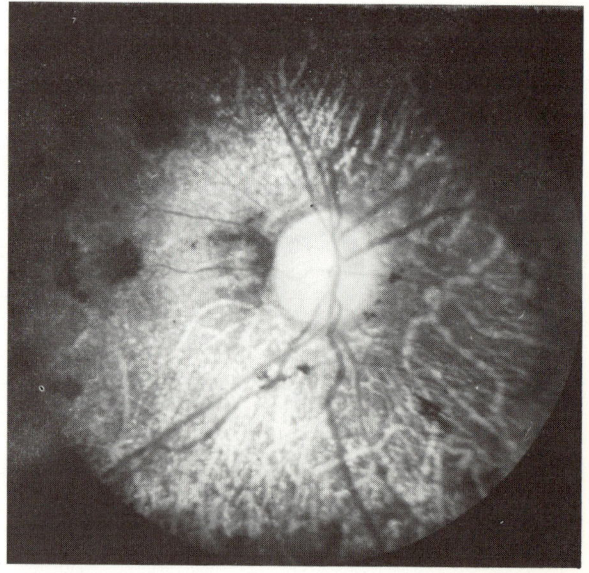

Plate 25 Posterior degenerative lesion of onchocerciasis (Hissette-Ridley fundus). Note healthy negro retina (upper right, dark sector), optic atrophy, choroidal sclerosis and clumping of pigment

death of a very few larvae in the choroid or the retina. The retinal pigment epithelium breaks up in this condition here and there, exposing the choroidal vessels. Small areas of choroidal sclerosis will be seen in varying degrees of advancement. These areas are bridged by healthy retinal tissue, although ultimately the latter will break down and the whole of the posterior pole may be exposed. Somewhere there is always a sharp, circumscribed edge to the affected part. Any one, or all, of the above changes may be found at any one time. In addition, several large pigment clumps are invariably found somewhere in the infected zone. 'Comma'-shaped pigmented structures are often present amount the pigment clumps, those being features which Rodger & Maertens (1977) suggested may conceal dead *larvae migrans*. More confusing still is the not infrequent occurrence of bone corpusculation, which is also discussed in Chapter 4. Bone corpusculation is far from being as common as believed. The author recently analysed one hundred of his old records and found that true bone corpusculation was present in association with a Hissette-Ridley fundus in only 7 per cent.

Treatment

During this period of time it is to be expected that in many of the nodules the adults will die and the nodules undergo fibrolipomatous degeneration. However, in a hyperendemic area new nodules continue to arise.

The best method of preventing the immediate risk of blindness is by removing the *mf. volvulus* from the skin by giving a course of diethylcarbamazine (DEC) in doses of at least 600 mg a day for 20 days. The reaction to this, as larvae already in the eye die, can be fairly well controlled by using mydriatics and steroids, although the reaction in the skin, which becomes highly irritable, is difficult to control. Antihistamines appear to have no effect. Antrypol (Suramin) is said to be effective in killing the adult worms and microfilariae, but this is not certain, and the drug, as it damages the kidney, has to be administered under supervision. No vaccine for diagnostic or therapeutic purposes has as yet been evolved, although this is under study.

THE DIAGNOSIS OF ONCHOCERCAL ANTERIOR UVEITIS

The terms 'granulomatous' and 'nongranulomatous'

'Granulomatous' uveitis is a term stressed and clarified by Woods (1961) to define a chronic, usually progressive inflammation of the uveal tract with active phases, a condition demonstrating a cellular infiltration, and followed by necrosis and repair, the latter being sometimes equally destructive. In the acute phase the infiltrate consists chiefly of monocytes and transitional forms of epithelioid cells. These cells, being adhesive, give rise to large mutton fat (lardaceous) keratic precipitates (KP); they also produce small nodules in or on the iris stroma and Koeppe nodules (or floccules, as they are sometimes called) at the pupillary margin, and adhesions between the back of the iris and the lens. Woods believes this form of uveitis results from active invasion of the uveal tract by live pathogens, *excluding only live larvae* (Fig. 3.14, 3.15 and 3.16).

The term 'nongranulomatous' uveitis is used to describe a nonpurulent inflammation of the uvea, in

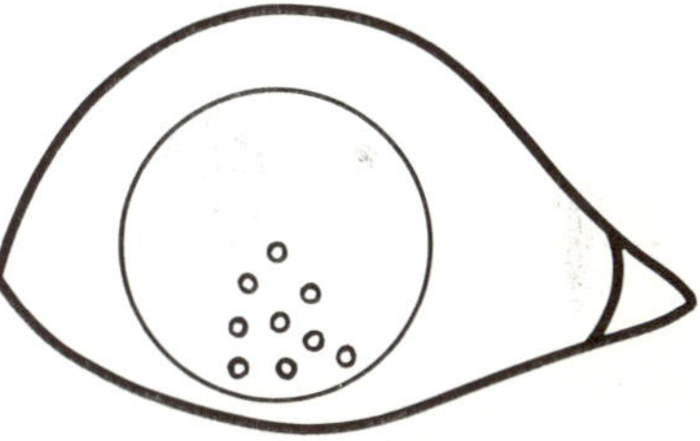

Fig. 3.14 Classic distribution of mutton fat (lardaceous) keratic precipitates (KP) on the back of the cornea (viewed directly) in granulomatous anterior uveitis

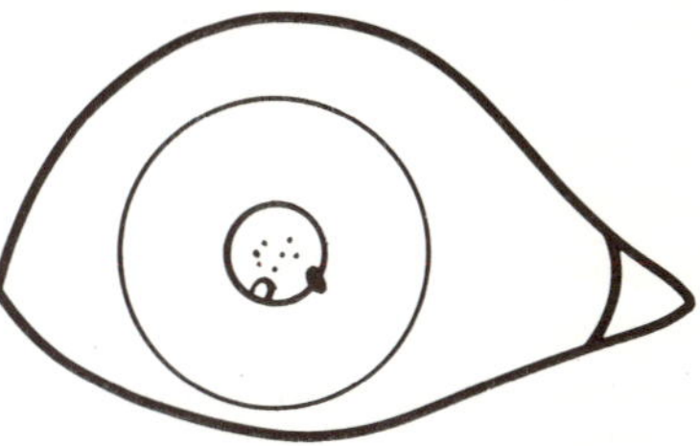

Fig. 3.15 Fine pigment particles on the anterior lens capsule and Koeppe nodules at the pupil margin, one pigmented, one not

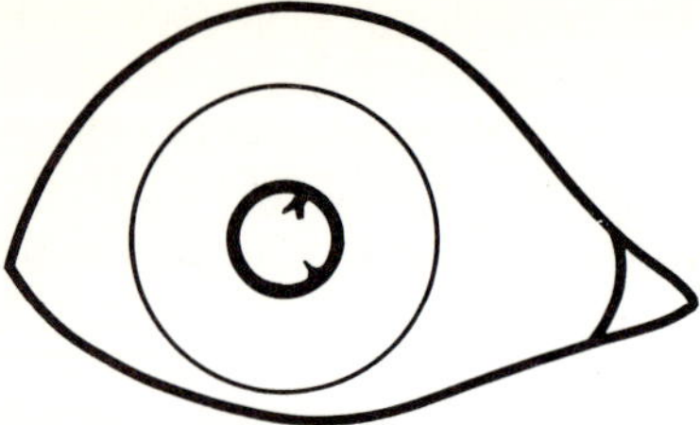

Fig. 3.16 Two posterior adhesions (synechiae) between the pupil margin and the anterior lens capsule

which the attacks are usually acute and self-limited, but often recurrent. The result is variable. Single attacks may subside leaving little or no damage. When severe and prolonged the damage may be as severe as in the late stages of a granulomatous uveitis. The infiltrate is of a nonspecific nature (small polymorpholeucocytes and lymphocytes). In consequence the KP are often small and coated with pigment (Fig. 3.17). Woods believes this form of uveitis is caused either by a rheumatoid factor, hypersensitivity (including larval), allergy (that is hypersensitivity to bacterial antigens), bacterial endotoxins, toxins of viral origin, or toxins from disintegrating elements such as the mf. of *O. volvulus,* or a mixture.

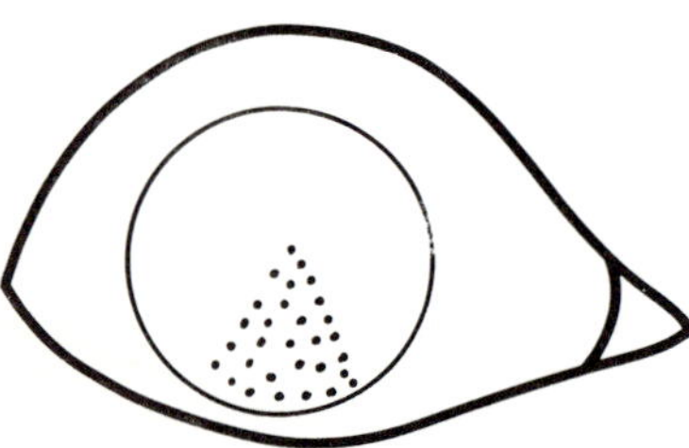

Fig. 3.17 Classic distribution of pigmented keratic precipitates on the back of the cornea in nongranulomatous anterior uveitis

A *mixed* uveitis can occur when the uvea becomes hypersensitive to the specific protein of a living pathogen—which has produced a basic *granulomatous* inflammation in the first instance—and then a later reinfection of the eye causes a superimposed nongranulomatous antibody reaction. While *mf. volvulus* live in remarkable harmony with man, even within the eye, the damage being done when the mf. die, endogenous invasion of the uvea by other living micro-organisms generally leads to a granulomatous uveitis, as in syphilis, tuberculosis, leptospirosis, trypanosomiasis, brucellosis and leprosy. On

the strength of the evidence, it is fair to conclude that Woods was right to decide that a granulomatous uveitis presupposes the presence of living organisms in the uvea and a nongranulomatous presupposes their absence, at least as a generality.

Epidemiological evidence

In the tropics, where an ophthalmologist usually works without much in the way of laboratory aid, it is impossible to diagnose with certainty the cause of an anterior uveitis, especially if seen in a late stage. A start can be made by determining if the uveitis is granulomatous or nongranulomatous, or both, and by marrying the clinical findings with the known epidemiologies of other uveal diseases. In a hyperendemic area of river blindness, for example, where onchocercal uveitis is nearly always nongranulomatous, where below the age of about 30 it is frequently not a severe nor even an acute condition, where above that age it only becomes severe in a small proportion of adults, onchocerciasis is the most probable cause.

The absence of the signs of acute granulomatous uveitis in hyperendemic areas of *river blindness* is well known and is illustrated by the findings of Rodger & Maertens (1977) in Zaire: out of 305 subjects all suffering from onchocerciasis, and none apparently from syphilis, tuberculosis or sarcoidosis, 34 exhibited small pigmented KP of nongranulomatous uveitis; lardaceous KP were present in 6; in 140 there were no KP of either type. Thus, when the end result of a non-granulomatous anterior uveitis is seen in a hyperendemic onchocerciasis area, it is quite reasonable to classify it as onchocercal on the basis of the epidemiological evidence, rather than as allergic or viral, or such. In the presence of a granulomatous uveitis on the other hand, one has to consider other probable infections, such as syphilis and tuberculosis, as well as parasitic diseases e.g. toxoplasmosis and sarcoidosis.

The histocompatability factor

A number of other diseases seldom diagnosed in the tropics, but known in Europe and North America to produce anterior and posterior uveitis, have to be considered (Brewerton, 1977). These diseases are largely nongranulomatous, but may be granuloma-

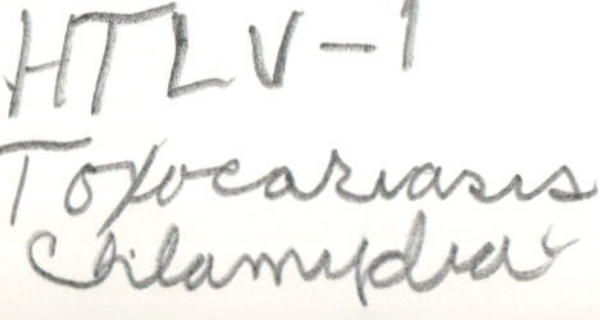

tous or even mixed, and include: *ankylosing spondyli-tis, sacroileitis, Reiter's syndrome, ulcerative colitis, yersinia* and *salmonella arthritis, Crohn's disease* without arthritis, *psoriasis* arthritis, juvenile chronic *polyarthritis* and *Behcet's syndrome.* Unfortunately, our knowledge of the frequency of the clinical nature of these diseases in the tropics is incomplete. The diseases most commonly associated with a nongranulomatous anterior uveitis from this list in the West are ankylosing spondylitis and Reiter's disease, not rheumatoid arthritis; in all three the inherited histocompatibility antigen, HLA B27 occurs, yet HLA B27 is said to be rare in Africans and uncommon in American Negroes. This may account for the low prevalence of spondylitis and Reiter's disease in Black Africa. However, the frequency and clinical nature of rheumatoid arthritis (of little interest when considering the diagnosis of anterior uveitis) is being increasingly diagnosed, especially in West Indian Negroes, so in the tropics it may very well be that ankylosing spondylitis and Reiter's disease have still to be fully recognised. They are not uncommon in Jamaica, where over 90 per cent of the population is African in origin, although Wilson & Graham (1979) state 'over the centuries a fair number of Caucasian genes may have found their way into the constitution of even the purest looking Negroes. In consequence there may well be important differences in the rheumatic diseases between populations of negroes in Africa and in the West Indies'.

Sarcoidosis

Sarcoidosis, which often exhibits a very marked granulomatous anterior uveitis, and a focal posterior uveitis can be difficult to diagnose. It is not transmissible by the usual methods, so Wood's theory that a granulomatous uveitis presupposes the presence of living organisms comes unstuck. The more usual belief as to the pathogenesis of sarcoidosis is that it is a paratuberculous disease, on the grounds that apart from the absence of caseation, the histological resemblance to tuberculosis is marked. However, there is also close clinical and pathological resemblance to berylliosis; this fact plus the lack of transmissibility previously mentioned has resulted in a third theory being put forward, and that is that sarcoidosis is a tissue reaction to an inert, nonspecific organic or

inorganic substance. The similarity to berylliosis may simply be a coincidence. Whatever its aetiology, the most important ocular lesion of sarcoidosis is an anterior uveitis, and for that reason it must be considered wherever such a condition is found to exist. The ocular change is characterised by discrete nodules which rise like tubercles in the stroma of the iris. They are somewhat larger and redder than a tubercle nodule, the blood vessels passing around the structure rather than through it, although this is hard to see in a Negro eye. The disease usually progresses steadily with short intermissions. Invariably, although not always, granulomatous, mutton fat KP, dense flare and Koeppe nodules are present as in all granulomatous uveitis cases. Posterior adhesions arise between the back of the iris and the anterior lens capsule from organised inflammatory exudate; because of these adhesions the pupillary margin is distorted and there may even be as inflammatory membrane around or over the entire pupil (Fig. 3.18). These signs are not specific. The posterior

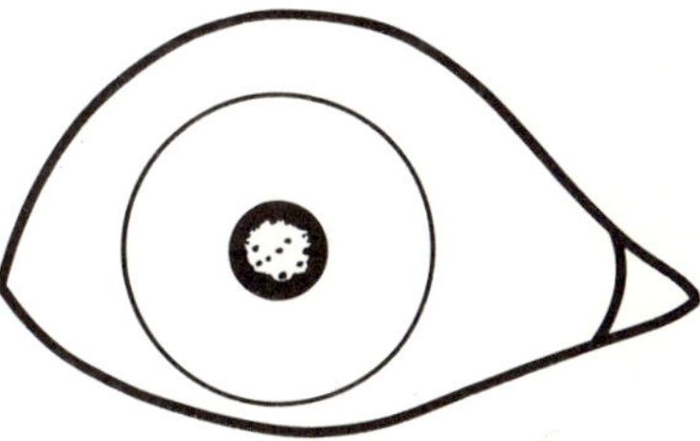

Fig. 3.18 Fusion of the pupil margin to the anterior lens capsule (seclusion of the pupil) by pigmented exudate in severe (plastic) anterior uveitis with pigment on lens face

uveal signs are less frequent, but when a sarcoid choroiditis (posterior uveitis) does occur, the lesions somewhat resemble those of miliary tuberculosis in size and appearance.

Gonorrhoea

One other disease must be considered in any discussion of anterior uveitis in the tropics, and that is *gonorrhoea.* Its effect on the external eye is discussed earlier in this chapter and on page 74. An endogenous anterior uveitis can occur in the course of a systemic infection by gonococci. The sequence of gonorrhoea arthritis and iritis has been frequently described in 19th century literature. The large proportion of the cases were males. The clinical appearance varies; one feature often claimed to be characteristic—although present in only about 1 in 10 cases—is where a profuse grey or yellow gelatinous mass forms in the anterior chamber, sometimes concealing the pupil, with or without a hypopyon or hyphaema. This gelatinous mass is not, unfortunately, characteristic, as at first thought, for it also occurs in onchocercal uveitis, and rarely in 'rheumatic' anterior uveitis, especially when butazoladine has been administered, unlikely in the tropics. In gonorrhea and 'rheumatic' anterior uveitis the gelatinous mass clears remarkably quickly, but in onchocerciasis it does not, and soon becomes fibrinous and white (flocculation). Gonorrhoea in the tropics is not as severe as in developed countries (compare syphilis) and an anterior uveitis seems to be excessively rare. It is possible, then, that many of the cases which have been described in the past are not gonococcal in origin at all although the bacilli are present, but are due to Reiter's disease, discussed with ankylosing spondylitis above. A history of anterior uveitis with urethritis, arthritis and (in half the cases) a raised ESR, without the complicating presence of gonococci, would clinch the diagnosis, but even when gonococci are present in the urethral discharge, although this is denied by some authorities, the uveitis may still be part of Reiter's syndrome. To date a gelatinous mass in the anterior chamber has not been associated with the latter disease, and so it is important to look for traces of such an exudate.

Other endogenous causes

Diagnosis of a uveitis (generally granulomatous) associated with the presence of systemic diseases (such as syphilis and brucellosis) depends in the last instance upon the clinical awareness of the examiner. Full clinical details are given under the relevant sections. If the primary disease is missed, there is little chance of identifying the cause of the anterior uveitis in a hyperendemic area of onchocerciasis.

LEPROSY

Natural history

Prejudice makes lepers the world's most common outcasts. There may be as many as 15 million lepers, 3 million in India alone. It is impossible to assess the number with seriously impaired vision. Lepromatous eye lesions are the worst, but are rare; the information we have suggests perhaps only 100000 have been blinded in this way. Tuberculoid leprous eye lesions are common, and it is likely that between 7 and 10 million people have ocular lesions as a result, an unknown number of whom become blind or part-blind in one or both eyes.

The mode of transmission is not understood properly, although it is generally admitted that transmission is from man to man. The responsible organism is *Mycobacterium leprae,* which in some ways resembles the tuberculosis bacillus. It is characteristically a slow replicator. This explains the long incubation period before clinical leprosy can be seen, often several years. No vaccine is available that is effective, but by the time this book appears, one might have been developed, as work has been going on for some time in an attempt to discover the immunological background without which the preparation of antileprosy vaccine cannot commence. In addition, attempts have been, and are being, made to perfect an improved diagnostic technique by means of a skin test by which clinical leprosy in doubtful cases can be more quickly uncovered.

The disease is distributed in a random fashion, principally within tropical and subtropical climates, in countries as vast as, and as thinly populated as, Zaire, or as vast as, and as thickly populated as India, or as small as Easter Island, an island belonging to Chile, and the only part of that country in which leprosy is found! There is no consistency. For example, there is less than one case per 100000 in Haiti and more than 10 cases per 100000 in the neighbouring parts of the same island, the Dominican Republic. Not only does the distribution of the disease exhibit great variety, but the clinical course varies a great deal. Untreated, the lepromatous form lasts for life, while the benign tuberculoid form tends to be self-limiting. In a large proportion of each there are serious complications.

In those whose resistance is poor (lepromin-negative persons), the phagocytic cells of the body ingest the bacilli, but do not destroy them and look foamy; these are classically known as *lepra* cells. In lepromin-positive persons there is good resistance; phagocytes (or histiocytes) destroy the bacilli and change into epithelioid cells. The clinical classification of leprosy depends upon the immune status, ranging from the tuberculoid form, in which the resistance is high, to the lepromatous form in which it is low. Luckily, the latter accounts for only one, or at most two, per cent of lepers in any endemic area. The accepted clinical classification is as follows:

TT   Tuberculoid
BT   Borderline tuberculoid
BB   Borderline, doubtful or both
BL   Borderline lepromatous
LL   Lepromatous

Development of the lesions

One is apt to think of leprosy as an infection with low invasive power, granulomatous in nature, a disease that can be localised or widespread, self-limiting or progressive. The fact is that even with a huge bacillary invasion (which is common) toxic absorption is absent, and that is its unique feature. Living bacilli in enormous numbers may cause little damage, apart from promoting spread (nasal swabs are the classic way of diagnosing and gauging the effect of treatment). When the bacilli die, cellular infiltration and oedema may surround them, as in the case of the microfilariae of onchocerciasis, and lead to local *granulomatous* damage; but the more serious immediate and later clinical consequences stem not from death of the pathogen but from the vigour of the cellular reaction at this stage. As only minute *strain* variations have been found, that is clearly not the explanation of the variability of the reaction. Within the body, the leprosy bacilli by both these means, by dying, or by producing an antigen-antibody reaction, can affect the eye, but principally involve the skin, joints and sub-adjacent blood vessels and peripheral nerves.

The skin lesions of tuberculoid leprosy are so-called because of the similarity to a tuberculosis pathology, namely the presence of giant cells, epithelioid cells, histiocytes and lymphocytes. It is generally not serious. The localised patches are usually dry and anaesthetic, and associated with nerve thickening, as the underlying nerves become involved. However, a reaction within the unyielding fibrous sheath of a peripheral nerve trunk may have irreversible distal consequences later, such as the wasting of muscles, like the orbicularis, which

guards the eye. This is even more true in the case of the borderline-tuberculoid type of patient.

Although the histopathology of tuberculoid leprosy resembles that of tuberculosis more than does the histopathology of lepromatous leprosy, the systemic changes in the latter are more closely linked with tuberculosis. Patients who are liable to contract lepromatous leprosy are also liable to contract tuberculosis, apparently because of a nonspecific group defect. There is, moreover, some evidence that patients who have had self-healing tuberculous lesions of the lung are less likely to contract leprosy than similar patients who have not had tuberculosis (Browne, 1979). Whatever the relation may be, the course of lepromatous leprosy is towards progressive involvement of the whole dermis by a continuous bacilliferous granulomatous process producing many surface nodules. Sheets of similar tissue may infiltrate anywhere. The consequent blockage of blood vessels and destruction of nerves with neuroparalysis leads to tissue breakdown with or without secondary infection, generally after 3 or 4 years. In the end, in these lepromin-negative persons gross deformities result, and although the condition may regress, it only too frequently leaves crippled, mutilated, ulcerating lepers, many of them blind.

Ocular features

Tuberculoid leprosy

Where the facial nerve is affected ectropion can result (Plate 26). Rarely it is bilateral. *Lagophthalmos*

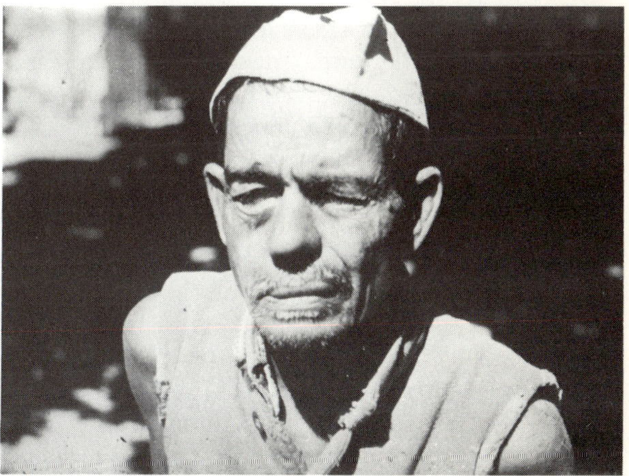

Plate 26 Facial palsy with resultant ectropion in tuberculoid leprosy

(inability to close the eye) is usually gross with consequent corneal ulceration. Where the tuberculoid lesion involves the skin of the lids, immobility can result in a pseudoparalysis, with loss of the eyebrows and lashes, and a deformity which either can result in entropion or ectropion (Plate 27). Apart

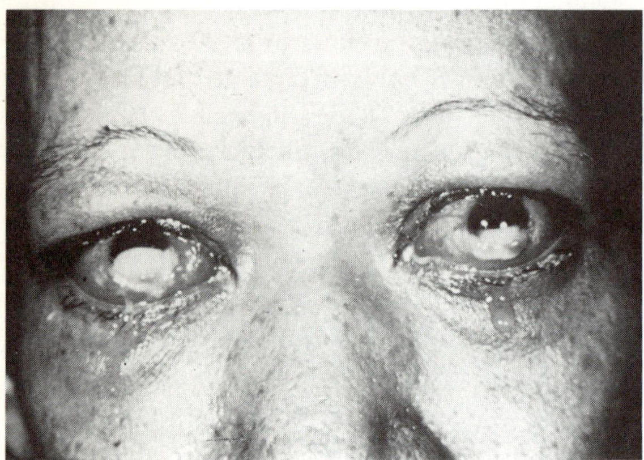

Plate 27 Bilateral paralysis of the lower lids with exposure of the corneas, ulceration and hypopyons in tuberculoid leprosy

from these mechanical changes, other ocular lesions are unlikely to occur in tuberculoid leprosy.

Lepromatous leprosy

Recalling that there are transitional changes between tuberculoid (TT) leprosy and lepromatous (LL) leprosy, the course of the latter is towards destruction of the eye. In borderline lepromatous leprosy (BL) you get the first evidence of the severe ocular changes, which reach a peak in lepromatous leprosy. A scleral nodule (leproma) may be seen as a presenting sign. This nodule grows and may develop into a sclerokeratitis, spreading across the cornea, and producing what is called a leprous hyperplastic sclerokeratitis. This lesion not only covers the cornea, but infiltrates the stroma as well. Such a lesion closely resembles the appearance of a benign mucous membrane pemphigoid lesion of the external eye. Another way in which the cornea is invaded is by subepithelial 'chalk grain' punctate opacities, which commence centrally at 12 o'clock, and with no real pannus lead to a subepithelial puntate keratitis in the upper half of the cornea. It can regress. Thickened corneal nerves and a thickening of Descemet's membrane are often seen associated with such an

SPK. The punctate opacities vary in size, but are usually small, and white (chalk grain), best seen by the slit lamp.

An interstitial stromal keratitis is common and results in many fairly large polymorphic opacities, but unlike that due to syphilis, vascularisation is not a feature, and if it occurs, it occurs late. The keratitis may be restricted to the deep layers of the stroma. It usually starts at the upper temporal quadrant, spreading to the upper nasal, then the lower temporal, and finally the lower nasal quadrant. This sequence is impossible to explain, but has been reported by many observers. The first opacities do not start at the limbus but a mm or so within. With the slit lamp they are seen as white or golden spots surrounding the corneal nerve fibres at several points. In short, the infection arrives in the cornea via the Schwann sheaths of the corneal nerves. The condition of stromal keratitis may progress to total opacification.

As for the uvea, the classic anterior uveal change is the 'pearl' a small clear leproma, a quarter of the size (or less) of the average Koeppe nodule seen in granulomatous uveitis. 'Pearls' can remain on the iris face for many years without symptoms. They occur singly or in a small group around part of the posterior part of the pupil, or even totally encircling it. They lie usually at the margin, or in the collarette area, and occasionally throughout the iris crypts. Sometimes they become pigmented, almost invariably so in the Negro eye (Fig. 3.19).

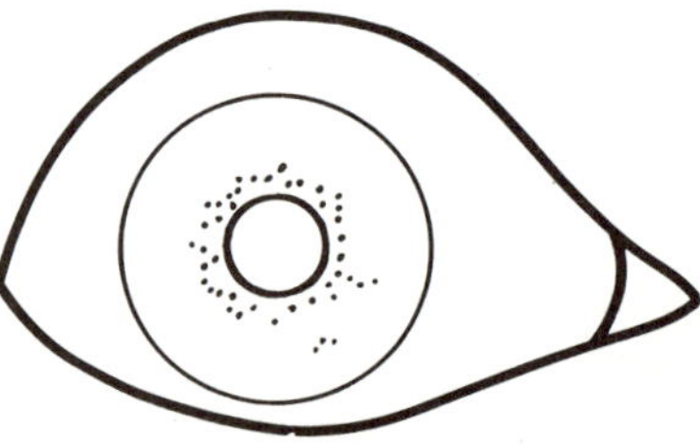

Fig. 3.19 Miliary pigmented leprous 'pearls' in lepromatous anterior uveitis

Acute mixed anterior uveitis may arise, with all the complications one associates with an untreated uveitis. It may be found in association with the interstitial (stromal) keratitis. The pupillary margin, as in any anterior uveitis, can be bound down by adhesions (Plate 28). A gelatinous hypopyonic mass in the anterior chamber has been reported, and may create

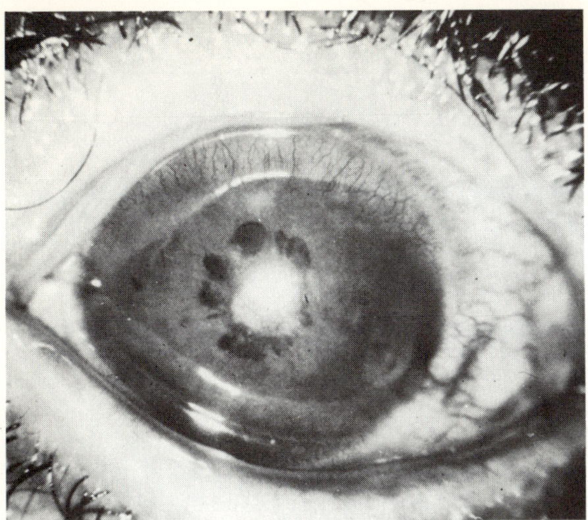

Plate 28 Lepromatous anterior uveitis with organised exudate covering pupil centre and a ring of posterior adhesions (scalloped pupil)

a pear-shaped pupil, similar to that found in onchocerciasis, and as rare. Deformed pupils often direct the attention to a past uveitis, along with such complications of untreated anterior uveitis as cataract or secondary glaucoma.

Although simple optic atrophy is described in the literature, it is not commonly seen, or perhaps one should say not commonly diagnosed, although there is no reason why it should not occur, any more than this disease should not affect the choroid and retina, where it has been equally rarely reported. Leprous 'pearls' have been reported in the choroid, pushing up the retina and looking like hyaline bodies, but never as the sole lesion. Choroidal 'pearls' have never been seen by the author, although he has examined lepers in leprosaria and camps in India and Africa for weeks at a time.

Treatment

Dapsone still forms the sheet anchor of leprosy treatment; this is an advanced sulphone: di-amino-diphensylsulphone. It is effective by mouth and generally well tolerated. However, it needs up to 10 mg per kg body weight per week (maximum daily dose 100 mg) over 2 to 3 years, or longer, to achieve bacterial negativity. Most patients in the East cannot afford to wait around for treatment over 3 to 4 years, for they depend on begging for a living, and as a result of interrupted treatments secondary resistance to Dapsone has been ever more frequently reported in LL and BL cases in particular. Lamprene (clofazimine 100 mg capsules) can be given three times a week in resistant cases; it is also a mycobactericidal and is safe and fairly effective at this level. Rifampicin is still under review, as are a few other drugs.

Dapsone resistance and toxicity occur in some cases of LL and BL leprosy. Acute inflammations in varying degrees of severity result, ranging from transient lesions of erythema nodosum leprosum (the lepra reaction) unaccompanied by constitutional disturbance to a generalised state of persistent tissue sensitivity that resists all treatment, even the use of large doses of steroids. Because the keratitis of leprosy is a tissue reaction to dead bacilli, it invariably becomes more active with systemic treatment and the same is true for a certain proportion of the anterior uveitis cases as well. Thus the eye requires constant supervision during therapy and topical ocular treatment with anti-inflammatory drugs may have to be employed.

Ocular onchocerciasis and ocular leprosy can occur together in the same eye, and, therefore, it is important in endemic onchocerciasis areas to make sure that both diagnoses are considered.

In the crusade against leprosy, primary health care is essential. India has developed rural clinics to implement surveys, education and treatment (SET). The aim is to reduce the prevalence by treatment, and correct physical deformities. Early detection and regular treatment are the goals, which is why the development of an antileprosy vaccine for both purposes is so badly needed.

Eye diseases commonly found in the tropics

The presence in developing countries of four or five of the severe blinding diseases in the world (discussed in Ch. 3) is to some extent balanced by the absence of several diseases common in developed countries. For example, retinal diseases, chronic simple glaucoma, optic nerve diseases and high myopia, which together account for 50 per cent of all blindness in the USA, account for perhaps only 15 per cent in the tropics; hereditary conditions have also been much less frequently recorded than in Europe or in Oceania.

Excluding the five blinding diseases categorised as major, the eye diseases set out in this chapter are considered to be those most likely to be seen in the tropics.

SWELLINGS OF THE LIDS

Swellings of the lids can occur with or without exophthalmos. It can involve one or both lids of one eye, or the upper lids (or both) of both eyes. The swelling may ulcerate or may not. In pigmented skin one of the cardinal clinical signs, *rubor,* is difficult to make out, so the patient's body temperature should be watched. Swelling of the lids of one eye due to primary infection, or secondary to infection, a tumour of the orbit, or of the eye itself, is fairly commonly seen in children and in adults in the tropics. A wide spectrum of pathological processes is involved.

Inflammatory lesions

Blenorrhoea of the new born
For description see Chapter 3.

Erysipelas (St Anthony's fire)
With so many facial infections existing in the tropics,

some common (e.g. yaws), some not (e.g. fungal infections), it is important to recognise the acute localised betahaemolytic streptococcal infection of the skin and subcutaneous tissue of the face, known as erysipelas. It may commence on or around the lids. It is characterised by redness, oedema and induration, and is associated with systemic symptoms, fever and prostration. The disease is very contagious. There is a clear-cut spreading margin, dotted with minute vesicles. The whole surface is shiny and dry as a rule. Gross oedema of the lids makes it impossible sometimes to view the cornea, but the latter is seldom if ever affected. There may be some oozing, particularly at the site of the infection, which is invariably a scratch or minute cut; ectoparasites should be sought. Treatment is with penicillin or erythromycin, either of which is more certain than the sulphonamides, and should bring the infection under quick control.

Lid abscess

Lid abscesses usually follow superficial infections, such as pyogenic infections of the lid margins and glands, usually with Gram-positive bacilli, although they may result from haematogenous spread from elsewhere, such as from the frontal sinus.

A lid abscess is treated as any other pyogenic abscess, with hot bathing, being incised only when it is well and truly localised and not hard. Erythromycin or ampicillin may need to be administered, and can abort it.

Acute dacryocystitis

Inflammation of the lacrimal sac follows pyogenic infections where the tear passage is blocked (usually between the sac and the nose). It may be blocked by a fungus (see Ch. 6), but more commonly it follows adjacent inflammation, sometimes within the tear sac itself. A large, inflamed swelling at the angle of the nose arises and causes oedema, congestion and closure of both lids. It is extremely tender to touch.

Antibiotics, as recommended for lid abscesses, are required in order to control the infection, and it may even be necessary to lance an abscess if one forms (Plate 29).

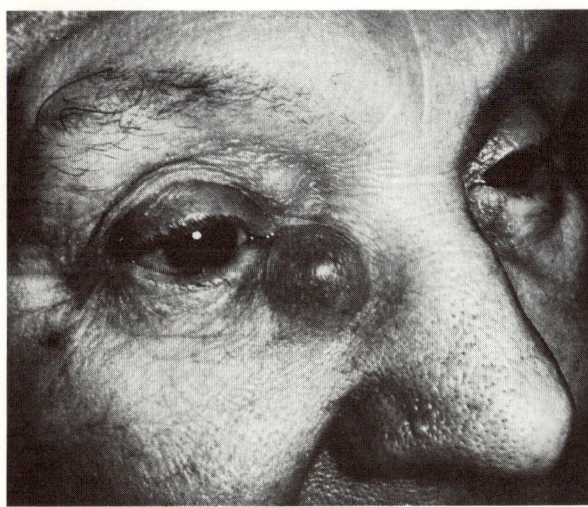

Plate 29 Abscess of Lacrimal Sac

Orbital cellulitis

The orbit is usually infected secondarily, either from the paranasal sinuses, usually by *Staphylococcus aureus,* or by haematogenous transmission, usually then by *Group A betahaemolytic streptococci.* Orbital cellulitis is more common in children than in adults. The fretful patient is ill, usually with slight fever and leucocytosis. The lids are swollen, red and oedematous. If an abscess is formed it can spread deeply and erode the bone. Thrombophlebitis of orbital veins going on to *cavernous sinus thrombosis* are serious complications. Then the fever becomes higher; there are rigors and oedema behind the ear, over the mastoid process; the patient becomes less active, maybe somnolent. *Cavernous sinus thrombosis* can occur without an orbital cellulitis as a primary lesion

following a blood-borne streptococcal infection, but this is infrequent. The lids in *cavernous sinus thrombosis,* although swollen, are not fiery; otherwise all the other signs of an orbital cellulitis are there.

Pressure on the optic nerve arising from a gross, untreated orbital cellulitis may destroy the nerve if it is not brought under quick control with antibiotics. Orbital decompression surgery may not be available.

Erythromycin or the penicillins are the best antibiotics to try, and should be given in large doses. If available, the cephalosporins may be needed if the patient is hypersensitive to the penicillins, or if the infection is known to be due to *Staphylococcus aureus* and/or Gram-negative bacilli.

Other (non-ulcerating) lid swellings

The following is a summary of the most frequent causes:
1. Calabar swellings
2. Lepromas
3. Dermoid cysts
4. Dracontiasis (in which several Guinea worms may be present at the one time)
5. *W. bancrofti* and *L. loa* adult worms
6. Cysticerci, which have been found in the upper lids in small masses
7. Neurofibromas (Plate 30)

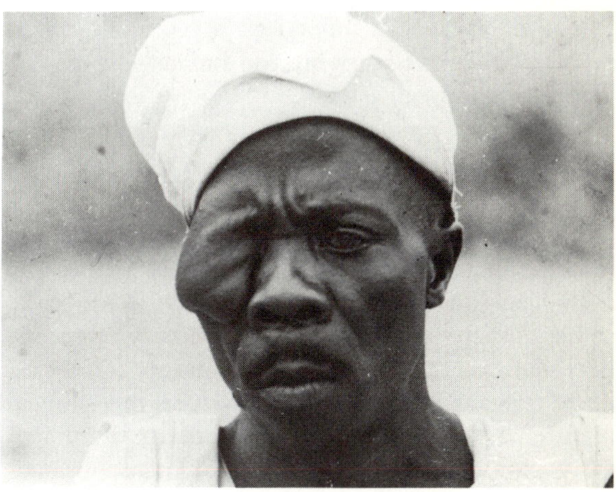

Plate 30 Neurofibroma of eyebrow

8. Sparganosis without ulceration
9. African trypanosomiasis involving the outer part of the lower lids

10. American trypanosomiasis involving the upper and lower lids (Romaña's sign)
11. Pseudoptosis in trachoma
12. 'Bung' eye in onchocerciasis
13. Lymphangiomas
14. Bilateral oedema due to allergy to ascaridotoxin
15. Bilateral oedema due to allergy to ancylostomo-toxin
16. Bilateral oedema during systemic invasion by the cercariae of schistosomiasis
17. Thyrotoxicosis (with exophthalmos) is rare, but not unknown in the tropics
18. Excessive SUVR, always binocular and lower lids (Ch. 2).

These conditions are all uniocular unless stated. They are described elsewhere.

Ulcerating lid swellings

The following is a summary of the causes:

1. Herpes simplex
2. Herpes zoster
3. Syphilis, primary chancre
4. Yaws, primary chancre or secondary sores
5. Leishmaniasis (oriental sore or espundia)
6. Lymphogranuloma venereum
7. Vaccinia
8. Squamous cell carcinoma.

These lesions are all uniocular. Mycotic infections involve adjacent tissues and do not usually pose a diagnostic problem.

Lid swelling due to underlying proptosis

Since the size of the bony orbit is limited, any increase in the volume of its contents pushes the eyeball and lids forwards. This is known as proptosis or exophthalmos. Many benign, primary or secondary malignant tumours, pseudotumours and developmental abnormalities may produce this clinical picture. In the tropics one has in addition to think of early paranasal and orbital fungal infections and parasitic infestations as well (see Ch. 6).

It is only possible in a book of this size—probably more helpful—to indicate those conditions that are most common. Congenital deformities are but rarely seen. Defects in the orbital walls, giving rise to cephaloceles (Plate 31) and meningocephaloceles,

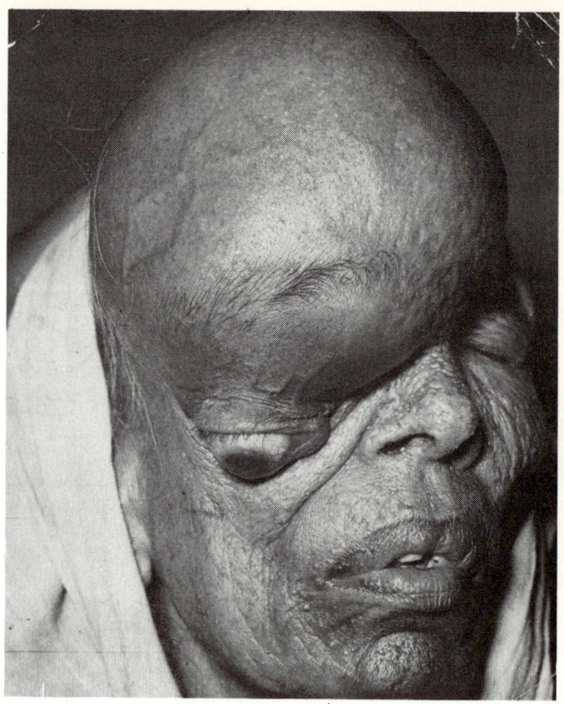

Plate 31 Anterior cephalocele

are even rarer than in developed countries, although a few cases have been reported from India and Pakistan. Congenital cysts of the orbit or brow, such as the dermoid, are remarkably infrequent, considering they are so common in the West. Congenital cysts and tumours in the upper fornix have been rarely recorded and are difficult to distinguish from parasitic and mycotic invasion.

There can be no doubt that retinoblastoma is common in Africa, although it is difficult to believe it is as common as the 'eight per cent of all blindness' reported in Malawi (WHO, 1979). This figure is probably due to the samples being far too small. Retinoblastoma is an inherited, highly malignant congenital tumour of the posterior segment in which both eyes are involved in about 30 per cent of cases. They are seen in infants as a lemon-coloured mass behind the pupil (Plates 32 and 33). 'Up country' in the tropics, without a doctor to turn to, these neoplasms push the eyeballs outwards and ultimately destroy them. After retinoblastomas, haemangiomas, mucoceles and chloromas are the most common tumours seen.

In the interior of Africa from 15°N to 15°S, and also in New Guinea, a highly malignant tumour

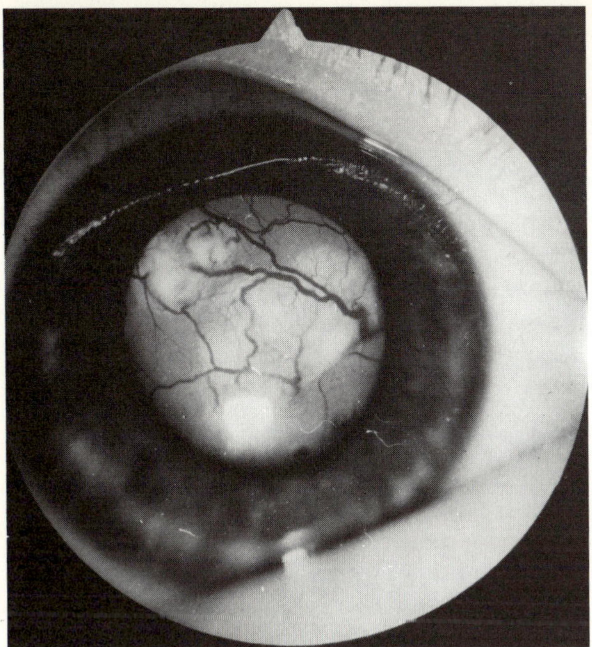

Plate 32 Retinoblastoma presenting behind lens

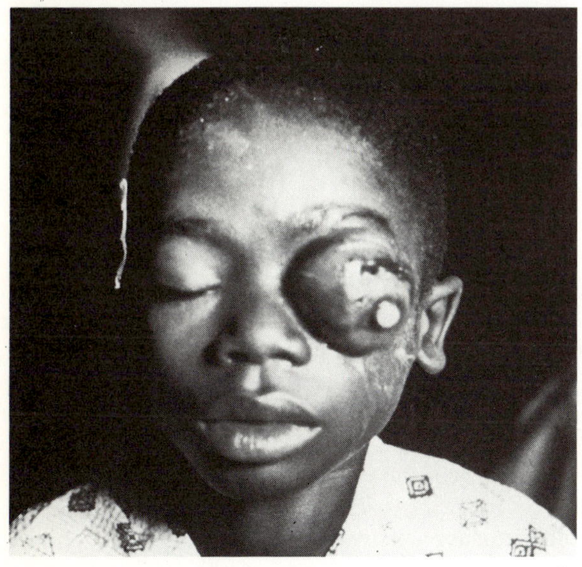

Plate 33 Retinoblastoma producing gross proptosis. The little boy died within six months

syndrome affecting children up to about 14 years is the commonest cause of unilateral proptosis in certain areas within these general areas. The peak age is said to be 5. It is a lymphoma known as Burkitt's

tumour, first discovered in Uganda. It is remarkably well tolerated until well advanced (Plate 34).

By far the commonest cause of lid swelling due to an underlying orbital lesion producing proptosis is a pseudotumour due to healed endogenous inflammation of the orbit itself (discussed on p. 51). Rare causes include glioma of the optic nerve, gumma and tuberculoma of the orbit, mycotic and parasitic infections, such as hydatid, sarcoma, endothelioma, neurofibroma and possibly sarcoidosis.

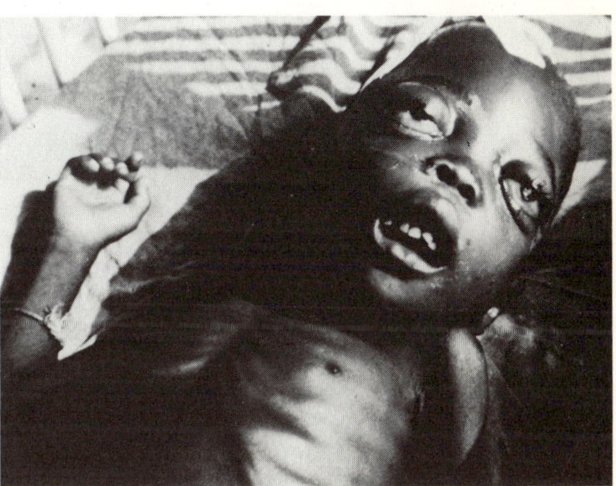

Plate 34 Burkitt's lymphoma (late stage)

The writer has seen a malignant choroidal melanoma in a Negro eye only once, never in an Asian eye; so at the least, one can say this tumour is uncommon in non-Caucasians, but they occur.

DEFORMITIES OF THE LIDS

In *entropion* the lid margins turn in, causing the cilia to rub against the globe. In endemic trachoma areas it is a common occurrence due to contraction of the scar tissue in the upper lid; in non-endemic areas it is much more common in the lower lid. Entropion is often a problem of the elderly, where chronic irritation may cause the lids to squeeze inwards constantly; the orbicularis muscle finally goes into spasm and the lower lid remains inturned, which results in trichiasis and corneal ulceration.

In *ectropion* the lid margins become everted, so that they no longer protect the eyeball. It more commonly affects the lower lids, again in the elderly, where constant mopping of the lower lids (as in the presence of lacrimation due to trachoma) drags the lids outwards. The exposed palpebral conjunctiva becomes hyperplastic and congested. It also occurs secondarily in granulomatous infections, and following paralysis of the orbicularis muscle (as in leprosy).

The treatment of these conditions is surgical and is described by Galbraith (1979).

ECTOPARASITES OF THE LIDS

Natural history

Lice and mites are widespread in the tropics. Infections by lice occur by close contact with verminous persons huddled together, especially during the cold wet season, or from infected clothing. Infections by mites arise from human contact with infected humans, dogs, cats and cattle.

There are three distinct subspecies of lice parasitic to man: *Pediculus humanus capitis* (the head louse), *Pediculus humanus corporis* (the body louse) and *Phthirus pubis* (the crab louse), which lives chiefly in the genital, inguinal and perianal regions. These infections are collectively called 'pediculosis'.

The follicular or mange mite (*Demodex folliculorum*) may be a true parasite in many or a saprophyte; it frequently comes from infected dogs, in which the same species causes mange. It is more common among house dogs in Asia than hunting dogs in Africa, although the latter live in closer contact with their masters.

The itch mite (*Sarcoptes scabiei*), the mite which causes scabies in man's skin, is also widespread in the tropics. Man rarely is infected by contact with animal scabies from dogs, cats and cattle.

With a magnifying loupe, the lice or mites should be sought on the eyebrows and eyelashes, and the ectoparasites (or their eggs) picked off and placed under a microscope for diagnosis. The largest is the female head or body louse (approx. 2 mm in length) with the crab louse next; mites are less than 0.5 mm in length. Body lice have smaller shoulders than abdomens, crab lice vice-versa. The itch mite is almost round, whereas the mange mite is banana-shaped.

Ocular features

Due to lice

Head and body lice particularly affect infants and children, the crab louse, usually adults. When the eyelids or eyebrows are invaded by the first two they attach themselves to the skin by their claws and lay their eggs (nits) on the eyelashes and body hairs. The scratching which results is largely responsible for the consequences, although it is thought that the excretion of the lice is an added irritant. Excoriation of the skin by the finger nails can lead to secondary infections and abscess formation. Although the normal habitat of the crab louse is the pubic and perianal region, they can also be found clinging to the eyelashes. Because of their tougher claws and sharper jaws the lesions produced are more severe. Irritation and pruritus involving the conjunctiva as well as the lids may be intense. Secondary infection affects the conjunctiva, a purulent secretion resulting, which sticks the eyelashes together. This appearance may suggest a secondary infection in trachoma. Abscesses of the soft skin of the lid, especially at the outer side of the eye, are not uncommon, and lice, or their eggs, should always be sought in such cases.

Villagers get rid of the scourge by rubbing the affected lids with wood ash. This removes the lice, but also leads to loss of the eyelashes (madarosis), leaving bare eyelids, swollen and inflamed. The appearance suggests trachoma, which, or course, may be present as well, further complicating the diagnosis.

Due to mites

Follicular or mange mites are known to invade man's eyelids and eyelashes (Rodger & Farooqui, 1959). Burrowing down into the follicles of the cilia and sebaceous or Meibomian glands, they group together in clusters, forming black pustules at the lid margins; occasionally a mite can be seen attached to an eyelash. Inflammation follows. As in the case of pediculosis of the eyelids, the damage is due partly to the activity of the parasite, partly to its excretion and partly to the host scratching himself. Even after the mites are apparently eliminated, a dry scaly, chronic blepharoconjunctivitis may persist, perhaps because of retained dead mites, or even the development of sensitivity, although this is not known for certain. Cases of severe chronic blepharoconjunctivitis should, therefore, always be examined for mites. The incidence is probably higher than we know, especially wherever dogs have a close relationship with man and canine mange is common.

The itch mite is, of course, much more widespread. The gravid female lays eggs in a burrow anywhere in the skin, including the eybrows. There are only a few records of scabies affecting the eyelids in adults, but it has been noted in children in association with conjunctivitis. The hatched larvae scratch their way to the surface and then pass down the nearest hair follicle, where they develop into adult mites; this gives rise to a scattered follicular eruption, which is extremely irritating. Scratching of the skin and secondary infection with impetigo or even erysipelas may result, and can confuse the issue. Scabies may also be confused with onchocerciasis where the skin can be extremely irritable.

Wherever you travel, scabies is usually known by a popular local name. In the UK it is known as 'the itch'. The sites of election in the adult are the fingers, hands, wrists, medial aspects of the elbows, breasts and genitalia. If these areas are found affected in association with encrusted eyebrows, the itch mite should be sought for in and around the eyelids, and suspect material examined under the microscope.

Treatment

All infections by lice or mites can be treated by one of several preparations containing dicophane and/or gamma benzene hexachloride. The hair, face (avoiding the eyes) and entire body should be painted with the emulsion, cream or lotion selected, and left for 24 hours before washing off; this should be repeated at least once more at 5 day intervals.

Where gross pruritus and inflammation of the eyelids remain, a topical combined antibacterial and steroid preparation, such as Aureocort (triamcinolone acetonide 0.1 per cent and chlortetracycline hydrochloride 3 per cent), can be used two or three times a day to the lids and their margins. Any coexisting conjunctivitis should be treated as well.

Proprietary preparations that are available include Esoderm (gamma benzene hexachloride 1 per cent and dicophane 1 per cent lotion), Lorexane (gamma benzene hexachloride 1 per cent cream) and Ascabiol (a pure benzyl benzoate 25 per cent emulsion).

SWELLINGS ON THE BULBAR CONJUNCTIVA

The four conditions to be described here must be recognised as what they are—minor changes which can be removed or left alone. As they may be confused with one or other more serious ocular lesions, their importance lies in the clinician being able to recognise them.

Pinguecula

Pinguecula is a common degenerative condition which occurs with age. It appears as a white, sometimes yellow, triangular patch situated on the bulbar conjunctiva along the horizontal meridian in the exposed interpalpebral area on one or both sides of the cornea. The lesion is said to be due to hypertrophy followed by degeneration, particularly of the elastic tissue. When small, the patches are usually round and white. The overlying conjunctiva is thin and friable. As it increases in size, it becomes polygonal and yellowish; this is due to a proliferation of elastic fibres. There is no fat in a pinguecula, despite its name, which suggests it. It is probably unrelated to pterygium and is without doubt not its forerunner. Sometimes small cyst-like cavities can be seen with the slit lamp within the pinguecular substance. The swelling does no harm, will never grow excessively and is best left alone.

Pterygium

Pterygium is caused by the growth or extension of the bulbar conjunctiva in the exposed area onto the cornea for reasons unknown, but believed to be long exposure to external irritants. A pterygium is wedge-shaped with the apex attached to the cornea. It is loosely attached to the cornea except at its apex where it is firmly adherent (Plate 35). It can be raised and a probe passed underneath the neck. Because of this fact, it may be that the pterygium commences as a degenerative process at the edge of the cornea and not in the conjunctiva. Its progression across the cornea is slow, but if untreated it ultimately will invade the pupillary area and lead to blindness. Both eyes usually are affected and sometimes at the 3 and 9 o'clock positions in each eye. Despite surgical removal, the recurrence rate is high in the tropics, and this is not wholly due to bad surgery.

A *false pterygium* is one where there is an adhesion between a diseased or damaged conjunctiva and the cornea. In it the conjunctiva is adherent throughout

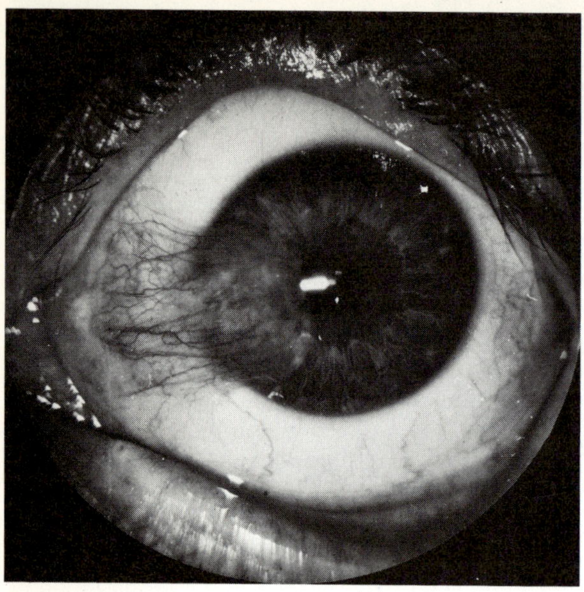

Plate 35 Pterygium

its whole length; there is no neck and no probe can be passed between the pseudopterygium and the underlying eyeball.

The treatment of pterygium is by surgical excision.

Lymphatic dilatations

A small clear swelling, or 'cyst' is sometimes seen on the exposed part of the bulbar conjunctiva. This is a lymphatic varix, or *lymphangiectasis*. It can increase or decrease in size, and is believed to result either from a local obstruction or from some form of irritation. As the causes continue, so the varices may multiply and become quite large. They give rise to irritation rather than pain. Examination with the optic section reveals the clear watery lymph contents and the absence of internal vascularisation. Sometimes a capillary network surrounds the lesion, or may even extend over the surface. If troublesome they are best excised without suturing, the area being touched with a cautery.

Nodular episcleritis

This is a fairly benign disease consisting of a localised nodular inflammatory patch under the bulbar conjunctiva, and once again in the exposed area, though not necessarily. It can be painful, is more common in women, runs a 6 week course or longer, and may occur successively in or around the initial focus.

Rheumatoid arthritis is a common cause in the over 40s, the systemic disease being increasingly reported from tropical countries. Allergies may also account for its presence, including allergy to tuberculosis. Metabolic disorders, such as gout, are also aetiological factors. The possibility of a nodule being an episcleral leproma or a parasite must be kept in mind.

Diagnosis is seldom easy. However, the average nodular episcleritis will yield to treatment with subconjunctival Depo Medrone. This is the treatment of choice.

Precancerous and cancerous changes

Elevated glistening white lesions surrounded with pigment are usually precancerous dyskeratoses of the bulbar conjunctiva (Ticho & Ben-Sira, 1970).

Flesh coloured or white elevations invading an arc of the corneal limbus are likely to be intraepithelial carcinomas (Bowen's disease). They are more common than in temperate climates.

Protrusive flesh-coloured invasive tumours in palpebral or bulbar conjunctiva may be squamous cell carcinomas. Total excision of the tissue is the only safe thing to do.

COMMON CORNEAL DEGENERATIONS

Arcus lipidalis

This is a form of lipid deposition in the peripheral cornea, generally associated with age. It appears as an opaque yellow-white arc or arcs, usually beginning in the lower or outer portions of the cornea; later these arcs may fuse to form a complete circle, which is separated from the limbus by a clear ring of superficial corneal tissue. This condition is also found early in life, and is then termed *arcus lipidalis juvenilis*. The so-called lucid interval between the edge of the arcus and the cornea measures up to a millimetre in width. As the condition progresses, the infiltrations—initially commencing in the anterior and posterior regions of the stroma—approach one another, producing an hour glass effect in the optical section, and later forming a solid, dense band involving the whole corneal thickness. Arcus lipidalis in the elderly has no clinical significance; in the young it is not frequently associated with one of the familial hyperlipoproteinaemias.

Arcus tropicalis

The author in 1959 observed and first reported the presence of an arcus which may in the tropics be confused with arcus lipidalis, or co-exist. The condition, called *arcus tropicalis,* was seen in all age groups. With the slit lamp the infiltration lies in the anterior stroma only. Moreover, there is no 'lucid interval' between the arc and the limbus; and it is generally found in the form of a complete circle. Histopathological examinations revealed that *arcus tropicalis* consists not of fats (although some fat was present), but of an infiltration into the superficial layers of the corneal stroma close to Bowman's membrane by chronic inflammatory cells. The infiltration is thickest at the limbal periphery, thinning out in the form of a wedge within a few millimetres of its passage towards the central cornea. The ultimate width corresponds to that of *arcus lipidalis,* that is a few millimetres. It is believed that *arcus tropicalis* results from limbal irritation in a dry tropical comate.

Band-shaped keratopathy

This is an important condition for two reasons, firstly because it must be recognised in order to distinguish it from climatic keratopathy; and secondly, because it is often indicative of a local or systemic disease. Its appearance at certain stages in its development is indistinguishable from certain stages in the development of climatic keratopathy (Ch. 2), but that they are two distinct clinical entities is certain when the histopathologies are compared.

In band-shaped keratopathy, a grey-white band slowly appears, starting at each side of the limbus, usually at 3 and 9 o'clock (Fig. 4.1). The affected areas extend inwards at a level slightly below the middle of the pupil until they meet in mid-cornea. The band does not have regular edges and nearly always exhibits dark 'holes', which are clear areas of cornea. Cytochemical staining reveals a deposit of calcium salts in the superficial corneal stroma early on, and later the addition of much hyaline degeneration. In climatic keratopathy the lesion commences as a faint

anterior stromal thickening; 'band' keratopathy works from the limbus inwards, but 'climatic' affects the entire diameter of the cornea simultaneously (more or less). Band keratopathy in the tropics invariably occurs secondary to chronic anterior uveitis, but it is known also to develop where there is hypercalcaemia, as in hyperparathyroidism, or vitamin D poisoning. It is known to occur in addition without any apparent abnormality as a *primary lesion* in otherwise healthy subjects.

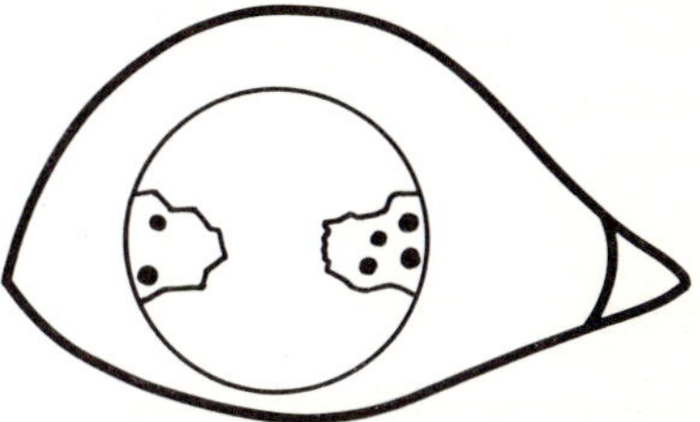

Fig. 4.1 Band-shaped keratopathy with black holes advancing across the cornea from 3 and 9 o'clock

Treatment by surgery or chelation is most unsatisfactory. If cataracts are removed, then the effect it has on a co-existing band-shaped keratopathy is to increase its rate of development. In the final stages there is never any evidence of the cysts which are characteristic of climate keratopathy and the latter unlike the former has an elliptical shape.

HERPES SIMPLEX KERATITIS

Natural history

The comparative infrequency of classic dendritic ulcers in Africa, Malaysia, Pakistan and India can probably be explained on the grounds that patients outside of the large towns are slow to come for treatment.

Clinically there are two types of herpes simplex virus: one causing genital infections, and the other most of the ocular manifestations, and infections in and around the mouth. In 1 to 3 year olds, it is the commonest cause of inflammation of the mouth, but it is rarely seen (even during fevers) affecting the eye. The primary viraemia with its buccal ulcers and fever in adult and child is self-limiting, lasting about a week. Subsequently, despite the presence of immune bodies, recurrent attacks in mouth, lip or eye are characteristic, especially liable to occur following minor injury (as by a foreign body), or when the resistance is lowered (as when following malaria, pneumonia or measles, hence the old term herpes febrilis). The high recurrence rate in the eye can make life a misery and lead to loss of sight. About one quarter of dendritic ulcers recur within 2 years, and of these 50 per cent within another 2 years. This trend continues. As minor injury can produce a recurrence, it frequently complicates the expected latency, so that recurrences seem more frequent. It must be stressed, nevertheless, that in the tropics, despite the existence of so many cases of fever, dendritic ulcers (and the aftermath, metaherpes) are seldom seen until late.

Development of the lesions

HSV in 90 per cent of people is ever present in the eye. It can be isolated from the tears and aqueous. External infections occasionally produce severe irritation as well as serious lesions, but generally there is no reaction. Viral replication within infected cells (when the viruses take over the metabolism of the cells) is the central event in the production of corneal epithelial destruction, giving rise to the classic branching (dendritic) ulceration; but this is not the only mechanism nor the only type of keratitis which results. Disciform keratitis and stromal necrotising keratitis, with or without an associated anterior uveitis, result from one of two complex cell-mediated immune responses, not yet wholly understood, and in many of the latter cases replicating virus is also present. Stromal abscess formation (keratitis profunda) is almost certainly associated with the presence of the virus.

Ocular features

The disease in almost any of its ocular appearances can spontaneously become quiescent, or persist and go on to loss of the eye. It can develop any of the various lesions described above in any particular order; thus disciform keratitis may slowly resolve, may become more inflamed, or it may move into the category of a necrotising stromal keratitis, or a new dendritic ulcer may be superadded, which readily becomes amoeboid or changes into an indolent metaherpetic ulcer with some stromal keratitis, or the lesions may simply never appear after the initial

dendritic ulcer has been cured. It is a confusing picture, difficult to assess, and unless caught early, difficult to treat.

Dendritic ulcer

Single or multiple (Plate 36), in one eye more usually than both, the small, branching figure is characteristic; it is not associated with underlying stromal disease. Its onset is as if there was a foreign body under the upper lid.

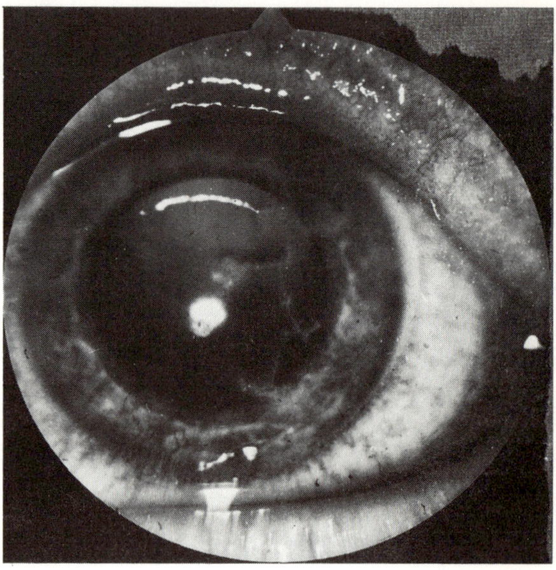

Plate 36 Four dendritic ulcers joined (unusually) together

Amoeboid herpetic ulcer

The untreated dendritic ulcer may enlarge to become an amoeboid ulcer. It can present at this stage, and because this stage is invariably associated with underlying diffuse stromal disease, which makes the entire cornea opaque, its nature may be missed.

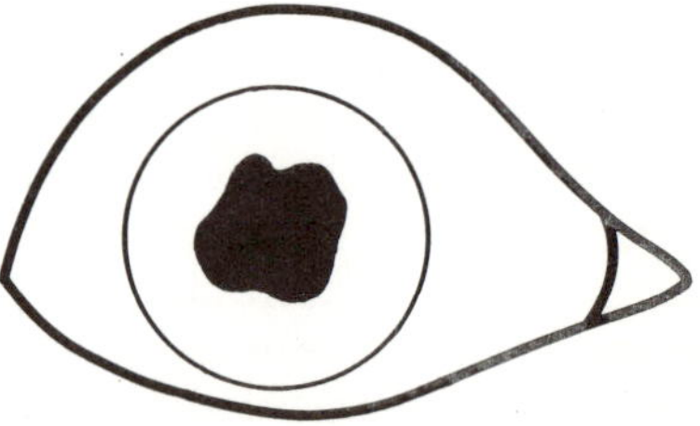

Fig. 4.2 Amoeboid ulcer staining heavily with fluorescein

Fluorescein staining will show up the stromal involvement, if the stain is left to soak in for a minute and then the cornea washed thoroughly. The amoeboid ulcer may then be made out (Fig. 4.2).

Metaherpetic ulcer

These ulcers are of two types: those which follow healing dendritic ulcers and those which follow healing amoeboid ulcers. In the former one or more minute round ulcers occupy the position previously occupied by the dendritic ulcer: they must be treated again. In the case of the latter there may be present one or two central islands of healthy tissue left over from the previous amoeboid shape, but these ultimately coalesce to form a large coin-shaped ulcer.

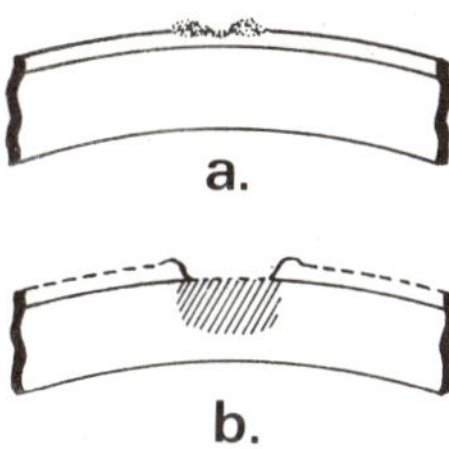

Fig. 4.3 Comparison between dendritic ulcer (a) and metaherpetic ulcer (b). The former stains with Rose Bengal and the underlying stroma is healthy; the latter is the reverse—the edge of the ulcer does not stain, but the stromal infiltrate does (from Falcon, Jones, Williams and Coster, 1977, Transactions of the Ophthalmology Society, 97, 348)

The significant feature is that in each there is underlying stromal necrosis and in the large ulcer in addition stromal lysis. Each arises because of damage to the basement membrane of the epithelium, which breaks down at that point. Metaherpetic ulcers have smooth, rolled rounded edges; the bases stain with fluorescein, and the epithelial cells at the margin do not stain with Rose Bengal. This is a distinguishing feature between a dendritic and metaherpetic ulcer (Fig. 4.3).

Disciform keratitis

As the name implies, the central portion of the cornea becomes occupied by a disc of varying relucency, visible to the naked eye; the loss of transparency is due to inflammation and oedema. In the optical section the disc is seen to be swollen; this is due more to oedema than to inflammation. A few

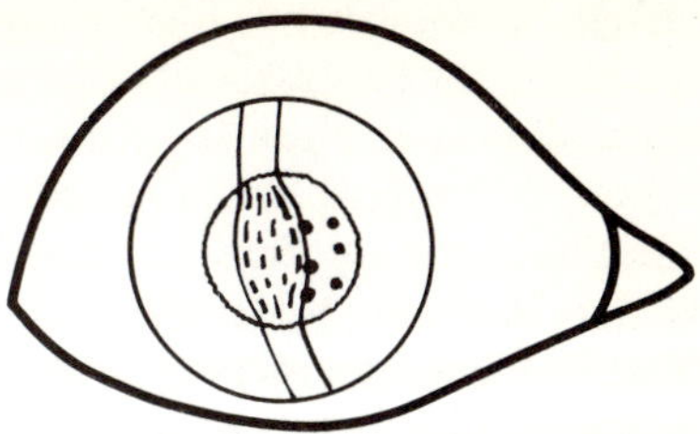

Fig. 4.4 Viewed directly, a circular central disc of semiopaque cornea with KP behind is seen in this composite diagram. The optical section is superimposed to show how oedema and infiltration thickens the disc

scattered, fairly small, lardaceous (mutton fat) KP can be seen on the endothelial surface of the disc, restricted to the area of the disc (Fig. 4.4). Unlike the stromal changes associated with amoeboid and metaherpetic ulceration, in which Jones et al (1977) have shown HSV replication in the stroma occurs, disciform keratitis is an immune response without any indication that HSV replication is involved in the abnormality.

Necrotising stromal keratitis

In certain cases intense neovascularisation of the cornea occurs. The high blood flow produces areas of epithelial oedema and stromal infiltration. There is frequently an associated wide ulcer, but not always. There may even be some anterior chamber activity due to an associated anterior uveitis, for example flare and 'star net' granulomatous KP.

In the centre of the swollen, oedematous and infiltrated corneal stroma, abscess formation may arise. Even at this stage recovery is possible.

Other signs of herpetic keratitis

So dramatic are the corneal cellular changes that it is easy to overlook other changes, such as the activity of

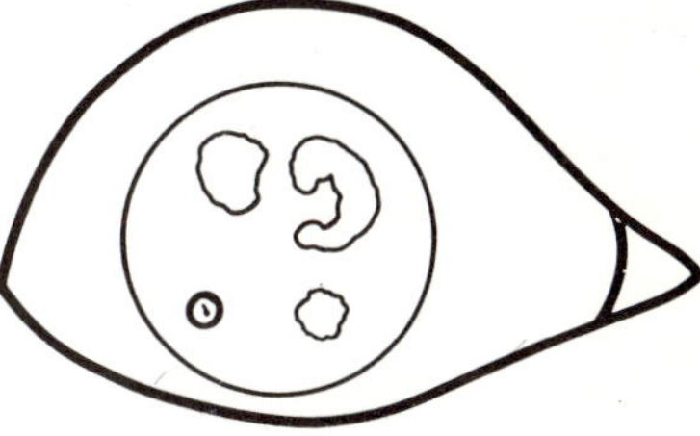

Fig. 4.5 Corneal scars, postherpetic, or following injury. The small scar (a nummular opacity) is nearly always the residual scar from a corneal foreign body

blood vessels. This takes two forms: either they are congested at the limbus, associated frequently with some oedema and perivascular infiltration, or new vessels grow in towards the affected part of the cornea. Similarly, the anterior uvea may be affected, either as a mild uveitis or as a severe uveitis with hypopyon. Residual signs include not only persistent blood vessels and evidence of past uveitis, but also scarring and deposits of lipids in such scars. These residual opacifications due to scarring and fatty deposits may be quite minor or extremely gross (Fig. 4.5).

Treatment

Debridement

When a dendritic ulcer arises the intercellular cement appears to have weakened, and so the affected epithelium is very loosely bound to the basement membrane. In consequence, debridement can be achieved extremely simply by wiping the corneal epithelium with a cotton-wool bud. Because the diseased cells can be removed so easily, this simple technique, used gently, separates them without any difficulty. The corneal epithelium is remarkable for the rapidity of its regrowth. It is important, despite this, to review the treated area every 2 or 3 days, because a considerable number of them reveal small ulcers, or even new dendritic ulcers fairly rapidly; in these cases it is recommended that debridement is carried out again, and the system continued as long as ulcers occur. It may be necessary to use Atropine and an antibiotic to avoid secondary infection, especially if recurrent treatment is found necessary. In recalcitrant cases, soaking the area in tincture of iodine after debridement may help.

Apart from wide debridement for dendritic ulceration, a small amount of debridement at the ulcer's edge may benefit amoeboid ulceration with stromal keratitis. It should not be forgotten that mydriatics and antibiotics to avoid secondary infection are appropriate in all these cases. These are frequently the only procedures open to one. Great care should be taken not to damage the stromal surface.

Use of anti-inflammatory and antiviral drops

Provided the epithelium is healed, or not involved, the customary method of treating a disciform stromal keratitis, or keratouveitis, is to give topical steroids, such as betamethasone, and a mydriatic. The least possible amount to control inflammation is advisable because of the side effects of steroids in these cases, which include not only stromal epithelial necrosis but also the risk of secondary bacterial or fungal infection, which is increased by the excessive use of steroids. Because of these factors it is wise not to use Betnesol drops more than three times a day in disciform keratitis and to reduce the application gradually to twice, then once daily, over 2 to 3 weeks, once the condition disappears. When steroid drops are unavailable, a subconjunctival injection of 0.10 ml Depo Medrone in the lower fornix should last 14 days, and be repeated 2 to 3 times.

The management of stromal herpetic eye disease with all the drugs available at the present time (Idoxuridine, Trifluorothymidine and Adenine Arabinoside at the same time as topical steroids are applied, prednisolone sodium phosphate 0.5 per cent and betamethasone sodium phosphate 0.1 per cent) is a highly skilled procedure, which, unfortunately, it is not possible to use in developing countries for the time being, by reason of the high cost. The co-ordination of anti-inflammatory treatment with antiviral is dependent upon the degree of inflammation in the corneal stroma and anterior chamber, and the presence and degree of corneal ulceration; it requires constant supervision in order to re-evaluate and modify the treatment (Jones et al, 1977).

HERPES ZOSTER OPHTHALMICUS

Natural history

A close relationship exists between the viruses of chickenpox (discussed in Ch. 5) and herpes zoster; it is probable that they are the same, though much remains to be explained. Both can cause chickenpox in susceptible contacts, although the risk is much less after contact with zoster. The opposite is not true; zoster has not been reported to follow close contact with chickenpox or other zoster patients.

When the herpes zoster virus involves the ophthalmic, first, division of the trigeminal nerve, it is called *herpes zoster ophthalmicus*. Typically, a vesicular rash on an erythematous base occurs along the first division of the fifth nerve. The eruption usually does not cross the midline. Stabbing pain may precede the rash by up to 48 hours. The skin of the nose is supplied by the nasociliary branch of the fifth nerve, and if vesicles are seen in this area of skin, then it is certain that the uvea will be involved, and due precautions should be taken. The ophthalmic nerve, giving rise to the frontal, sends fibres over the eyelids onto the external ocular membranes, which will also be affected by the eruptions. The disease usually occurs in those (whose immunological mechanisms are run down), who have been in contact with youngsters suffering from chickenpox.

The diagnosis is made on clinical grounds.

Ocular features

The bulbar conjunctiva and the corneal surface are always affected. There is some bulbar congestion with corneal anaesthesia (which seldom fully recovers), and the discrete subepithelial corneal infiltrates, which arise, and involve the anterior substantia propria, later become erosions; they seldom become secondarily infected. The infiltrates sometimes progress in the opposite direction into the deeper layers of the cornea and folds can appear in Descemet's membrane. When the nasociliary branch is involved, then there is an associated anterior uveitis, which may be a mild nongranulomatous one, but can also be severe with mutton fat KP, posterior synechiae and even a hypopyon. It can then become a long intractable, painful condition, not infrequently complicated by secondary glaucoma. Hypopyon is said to be a more frequent complication than glaucoma, but this is not the author's experience. Motor palsies involving the extraocular muscles, a haemorrhagic retinopathy and optic neuritis have also been described as rare complications. It is a distressing disease with persistent forehead paraesthesia. It may be accompanied by a corneal infection with *herpes simplex virus*.

Treatment

If a case presents with the side of the nose involved, but before the anterior uveitis arises, it is as well to dilate the pupil and give Diamox night and morning as a preventive measure against iris adhesions and secondary glaucoma. If steroids are available they do not harm the corneal erosions, although the cornea must always be watched closely. It is important first to exclude the existence of dendritic ulcers, rare though their association is. The external ocular lesions should be treated with an antibiotic ointment to prevent secondary infection. This is about all one can do, although there is a school of thought which says that the sooner large doses of systemic steroids are given the better. If this drug is available, then the best treatment is to give 20 mg prednisolone t.d.s. for 3 days, 15 mg t.d.s. for 3 days, 10 mg t.d.s. for 6 days and 5 mg t.d.s. thereafter, gradually fading it out over 3 to 4 weeks. During this period of time, if the patient's general condition deteriorates, then it may be there is an underlying pneumonitis which is being obscured by the systemic steroids, and the latter should be discontinued; this is a not uncommon happening in tropical countries in the elderly.

The clinical manifestations of zoster have in the past been divided into two types, the viral and the symptomatic. The second aetiology is questionable. It is based on the assumption that the ophthalmic root of the trigeminal ganglion is involved *secondarily* in some infective, neoplastic or traumatic disturbance, such as syphilitic or tubercular meningitis or lymphatic leukaemia. In other words, this kind of ophthalmic zoster is regarded as essentially a neuroparalytic keratitis.

GLAUCOMA

Natural history

The aqueous humor is both a secretory product and a filtrate, and is formed by the ciliary processes behind the iris; it passes through the pupil into the anterior chamber, and out through the spongy tissue (trabecular spaces) where the cornea joins the periphery of the iris. Once through the trabecular spaces, the aqueous passes into a circular canal (Schlemm's)—external to the corneal limbus and within the sclera. It finally escapes through holes in the canal into the external veins of the eyeball via aqueous veins (that is, veins in which aqueous and blood mix), and returns to the general circulation.

In glaucoma, somewhere along the line, the outflow of the aqueous becomes inadequate and the intraocular pressure rises, thereby damaging the retina and the optic nerve.

The following is a simple but practical classification of glaucoma related to the investigatory facilities of the geographical regions with which we are concerned;

1. Primary glaucoma
   a. Primary open angle glaucoma (chronic simple glaucoma, wide angle glaucoma, glaucoma simplex)
   b. Primary narrow angle glaucoma (closed angle glaucoma)
2. Congenital glaucoma
   a. Infantile
   b. Juvenile
3. Secondary glaucoma
4. Absolute glaucoma

These various types of glaucoma are found in all countries of the world. A dominant form of inheritance, regular and irregular, has been well recorded in the case of the non-infantile primary glaucomas; the penetrance is higher in narrow angle glaucoma than in open angle. The primary glaucomas are also closely related to the inheritance of susceptibility to steroid-induced raised ocular pressures. In addition, it has been claimed that about 10 per cent of all primary glaucoma patients have poor glucose tolerance, or are overtly diabetic.

Ocular features

Primary open angle glaucoma

It is not easy to plot visual fields in unsophisticated peasant-farmers, who speak a local dialect. This is unfortunate, as perimetry and scotometry are great diagnostic aids, for example in deciding whether a patient has ocular hypertension where there is no field loss and no cupping. Perimetry may be attempted by using Traquair targets against a dark background; but at the best it can only give a rough idea of field changes, hard to identify as characteristic of glaucoma. Thus, the clinician is at a great disadvantage in the tropics.

Gonioscopy is a simple procedure and will separate a primary open angle glaucoma from a primary narrow angle (subclinical) glaucoma, for in the former the filtration angle is wide and free of abnormal mesodermal cells, although in pigmented races some pigment is generally present. An open angle is unobstructed by the root of the iris. The technique is described in Chapter 1.

Intraocular pressures above or equal to 21 mm Hg, whether using an indentation (Schiotz) or applanation tonometer, are suspicious; pressures above or equal to 24 mm Hg are highly suspicious of glaucoma. There is a great variance in intraocular pressures in borderline cases, in whom tensions may have returned to normal by the time the patient is examined.

The fovea is the last part of the retina to be damaged by elevated ocular pressures, so visual acuity may be excellent even when the disease is far advanced and the visual fields grossly shrunken.

The differential diagnosis of optic atrophy with or without cupping of the optic nerve head is discussed in the section on 'The problem of optic atrophy' later in this chapter, which should be read in conjunction with the present section. The diameter of the cup divided by the diameter of the disc in primary open angle glaucoma is generally 0.3; the more the C/D ratio exceeds 0.3 the more likely it is that one is dealing with a chronic open angle glaucoma (Plate 37).

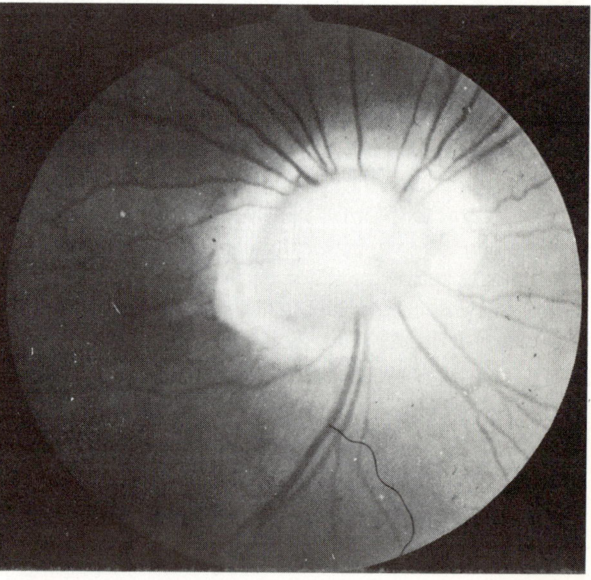

Plate 37 Optic atrophy with cupping in chronic open angle glaucoma

Open angle glaucoma is usually symptomless. In advanced cases there may be blindness in one eye, but not in the other. Diagnosis has to be made in the field or small unit with the ophthalmoscope, tonometer and gonioscope.

Primary narrow angle glaucoma

Usually, when there is a high intraocular pressure (IOP) there is an extremely painful eye, which brings the patient to the clinic in quick time. The eye is acutely congested; the acute phase can affect one or both eyes simultaneously. Pressures can range from 30 to 100 mm Hg.

Gonioscopy often reveals a slightly open, if narrow, angle, when the pressure is within normal, but a closed angle when raised. The iris in these patients, even when the tension is not raised, arches forwards and the anterior chamber is shallow in consequence. These features are exaggerated when the intraocular pressure is great. The fluctuations in IOP are more marked and the range far wider than in primary open angle glaucoma. Acute elevations of ocular pressure may be so high (100 mm Hg) that the perilimbal capillaries are compressed and diffusion of fluid into the cornea, especially epithelium, is slowed down; corneal oedema results. This gives rise to vivid haloes (coronas) around lights. Vision is blurred and there is severe ciliary neuralgia and headache. The slowing of the blood flow affects the outer and inner vasculature of the eyeball as well as the cornea. The eye is markedly congested. Protein and cells increase in the aqueous, simulating an anterior uveitis. Under constant high pressure the pupil is unable to contract and remains in a semi-dilated state. The patient may vomit with the pain.

The basic mechanism would appear to be a relative pupillary block with the lens acting as a 'plug' to the pupil (Miller, 1977). The same author states that primary narrow angle glaucoma in a Negro tends to be chronic. If true, it must be a genetic phenomenon (see later in this chapter). In South East Asia primary narrow angle glaucoma is more common than in the West, but it is still not as common as primary open angle glaucoma.

Congenital glaucoma

This condition is due to malformation of the filtration angle and is characterised in the infant child by a deep anterior chamber, usually an enlarged cornea and later by ruptures in Descemet's membrane. It is inherited as an autosomal recessive. Surgical treatment must be carried out by an experienced eye surgeon, the sooner the better.

Secondary glaucoma

Secondary glaucoma arises in consequence of another recognisable ocular disease, such as inflammation of the anterior uvea, central retinal vascular block, the presence of intraocular *mf. volvulus* with anterior chamber activity (perhaps), injury, pupillary block by a vitreous 'plug' after cataract surgery, or rarely, in association with an intraocular tumour. In such cases, especially in a severe anterior uveitis, it is very easy to forget about the intraocular pressure. *Secondary glaucoma is extremely common in tropical ophthalmology, where so many acute eye diseases remain untreated.*

Absolute glaucoma

This term refers to an eye in which the pressure has risen irreversibly,. It is invariably a blind eye. Excision of the eye is the only really effective treatment, although pain may be controlled by retrobulbar injections of 0.5 ml of 2 per cent lignocaine followed down the same needle by 1 ml of 40 to 90 per cent alcohol. Absolute glaucoma is not uncommon where a postthrombotic glaucoma has developed, or where postinflammatory pupillary block has existed for some time. Central retinal venous thrombosis is uncommon in most developing countries.

Treatment of glaucoma

Urgent treatment is required for an acute narrow angle glaucoma. It should be controlled first by giving Diamox 500 mg by mouth (or intravenously) and 250 mg Diamox tablets every 6 hours thereafter, each with one or two tablets of Slow K (which makes good the potassium loss induced by Diamox, a diuretic). Simultaneously, topical treatment with meiotic drops such as 1 to 3 per cent Pilocarpine is needed to draw down the iris and open up the angle. This is not the only effect pilocarpine has in lowering the pressure. In prolonged cases there may be no response by the pupil even when pilocarpine 3 per cent is given every few minutes for half an hour, every 15 minutes for 2 hours, and then hourly till next morning. Pilocarpine drops q.d.s. should be instilled into the unaffected eye as a precaution for several more days.

Surgery is the ultimate treatment for narrow angle glaucoma, but the operation is less likely to give trouble if the intraocular pressure is lowered beforehand, preferably within 24 hours. Surgery in an interval between acute attacks, while pilocarpine 1 per cent is instilled once or twice daily, especially at night, is the ideal. Repeated acute and subacute attacks of narrow angle glaucoma will in the end damage the drainage channel so that an acute-on-chronic-on-acute condition can result. On the other hand, moderately high intraocular pressures may be recorded in chronic simple glaucoma where the angle is open, but not fully wide (say, 30 mmHg). When the pressure is high and the cornea steamy, it is impossible to use the gonioscope and, therefore, impossible to diagnose the width of the angle; in such cases it is wiser to carry out a drainage operation rather than a simple peripheral iridectomy.

The operation of choice for chronic open angle glaucoma is trabeculectomy. However, it may be kept in check with medical treatment, using varying strengths of pilocarpine three or four times daily, with or without a Diamox Sustet (500 mg slow release) in the evening, with or without an additional Diamox tablet (250 mg) at noon, each given with a Slow K tablet, preferably. The prolonged use of any medicament in developing countries is unlikely to be successful because of lack of co-operation and the cost of the drugs involved in lengthy treatments. Moreover, the expense of other, more successful, antiglaucoma drops such as Timolol 0.5 per cent bd and Eppy 1 per cent b.d. with or without Diamox is also ruled out. In short, surgery is the more practical answer.

Note. Use of topical steroid eyedrops will be restricted to a few people only in developing countries due to the high cost, but as inferred in the opening paragraphs, many non-infantile glaucomas (which may be unrecognised or dormant) inherit a susceptibility to steroid-induced raised intraocular pressure, so that where treatment with topical steroids is being carried out, the intraocular pressures will rise. These patients should be treated as open angle glaucomas and the steroids discontinued.

RETINAL BONE CORPUSCULATION AND THE QUESTIONS IT POSES

Primary retinitis pigmentosa

In endemic areas of onchocerciasis, in regions of the world where syphilis is still present and where viral diseases such as measles still reach epidemic proportions, it is vital to distinguish primary retinitis pigmentosa from pseudoretinitis pigmentosa. Although the former exhibits a variety of inherited patterns, it is most frequently seen in developed countries as a simple recessive trait; nevertheless, it has a dominant and sex-linked transmission as well, so that where consanguinity occurs, as in high caste Moslem and Hindu communities, where cousin marriages are common, a marked increase in the prevalence rate is found. This social background in itself is an aid to its diagnosis. Sex-linked transmission is the most difficult to diagnose, for it can be uniocular and assume different forms, some of them resembling, for example, the pigmentary corpusculation which follows blockage of a retinal branch artery. Males are more likely to suffer from primary retinitis pigmentosa than females owing to the occurrence of sex-linked cases. The condition is generally bilateral, which may not be the case in pseudoretinitis pigmentosa.

The condition begins at adolescence with night blindness; although the patient may not admit it, the minimal light threshold is always poor. Ophthalmoscopic findings may be absent for several years, but they inevitably become obvious. At first, the retinal pigment epithelium degenerates, the pigment migrates and adopts the shape of bone corpuscles, scattered throughout the periphery. They lie preferentially alongside the blood vessels, on some of which they form short sheaths or cuffs. The process spreads both centrally and peripherally until the choroidal vessels are exposed; but the latter are not usually sclerosed, although, to complicate matters, a second mutation producing choroidal sclerosis may occur with primary retinitis pigmentosa. As the disease advances the retinal arteries become thin and straight, and the optic nerves pale or waxy. In the final stages posterior polar cataracts not infrequently develop and macular degenerations are also seen, although somewhat rarely. Myopia is not infrequently associated with this condition and may be severe.

Rubella

It is noted in Chapter 6 that rubella can produce a secondary retinitis pigmentosa among other embryopathic lesions, but as it is so very common in outlying tropical districts, few if any mothers have not contracted rubella prior to pregnancy, with the result that the classic rubella lesions are seldom, if ever, seen, except in migrants.

Measles

In the case of measles, a neuroretinitis, followed by a slowly developing secondary pigmentary degeneration, occurs in children, rarely in adults, following the acute phase. When this is seen in later life, it poses a problem of diagnosis. As in syphilis, measles is not infrequently associated with pigmentary macular changes following oedema during the acute phase. This association in the case of primary retinitis pigmentosa is rare. Although measles may simulate classic retinitis pigmentosa, it not infrequently presents as an atypical pigmentary degeneration, comparable to the various appearances X-linked primary degenerations demonstrate.

Syphilis

Certain ocular changes in syphilis somewhat resemble primary pigmentary degeneration of the posterior segment. They are described on page 86, but are summed up here.

In congenital cases the 'pepper and salt' fundus should not be confused with the bone corpusculation under discussion nor should the scattered peripheral retinal scars sometimes found in congenital lues, as bone corpuscle forms are absent. However, a congenital syphilitic pseudoretinitis pigmentosa, which closely resembles the real thing is also seen, if rarely. In the latter other signs of congenital syphilis will be present, as may signs of quiescent anterior uveitis.

In acquired syphilis in the late secondary or early tertiary stages, a peripheral secondary pseudoretinitis pigmentosa can occur. This also is a difficult one to diagnose. It may follow an initially diffuse neuroretinitis which tends to affect the optic nerve and the area around the optic nerve, and yet at the same time leads to the development of peripheral bone corpusculation.

The most common manifestation of all is disseminated chorioretinitis. The changes are widespread and always involve the posterior pole. The dispersal of pigment is so gross and closely bound with choroidal scars that there should be no question of confusing it with a primary retinitis pigmentosa, but in onchocerciasis areas it does confuse the diagnosis. The ocular pigment being so dense in the Negro eye there is quite frequently a violent peripheral reaction with marked bone corpusculation. This is more gross than in any other pigmentary degeneration. In about half the cases only one eye is involved. Usually there is white sheathing of one or more central vessels, and there may be a few haemorrhages. Sheathing occurs in the posterior degenerative lesion of onchocerciasis, but it is not as common and occurs on the vessels close to the disc; and there are no haemorrhages. These are helpful subsidiary features where dense bone corpusculation is found.

In an endemic yaws area, which frequently coincides with hyperendemic onchocerciasis, venereal syphilis is uncommon and may be excluded on epidemiological grounds unless the clinical picture is highly suggestive. In the absence of yaws, but in the presence of endemic syphilis, the possibility that a few cases of venereal syphilis might occur must not be forgotten.

Onchocerciasis

The onchocerciasis fundus associated with a pseudoretinitis pigmentosa invariably exhibits somewhere a sharp demarcation between healthy retina and that part of it from which the retinal pigment epithelium has been, or is being, removed; the syphilitic does not. Secondly, as mentioned above, the bone corpusculation is not nearly so dense as in the pseudoretinitis pigmentosa associated with a disseminated syphilitic neuroretinitis; thirdly, central pigmentary clumping in onchocerciasis, although more gross than in primary retinitis pigmentosa, is not as gross, nor are the clumps as scattered, nor as numerous, as in syphilis; fourthly, in onchocerciasis one at least of the pigment clumps is likely to be 'comma' shaped; most of them round. This is never seen in syphilis. Lastly, it is to be remembered that in a hyperendemic area of onchocerciasis only about 10 per cent of posterior degenerative lesions exhibit bone corpusculation: the dominant fundal picture is one of choroidal sclerosis. The latter is not found in syphilis. Although it can occur as a second associated mutation with primary retinitis pigmentosa, it is not so common, whereas in onchocerciasis choroidal sclerosis is the rule. In essence the diagnosis of the posterior degenerative lesion of onchocerciasis (as distinct from an onchocercal posterior chorioretinitis) may fairly be said to be based on two factors: the close epidemiological association (and its absence from adjacent areas where onchocerciasis does not exist) of the so-called Hissette-Ridley fundus, and the fact that consanguinity is taboo in most tropical countries, which makes the high prevalence rate of this lesion unlikely to be related to hereditary retinitis pigmentosa and choroidal sclerosis, at least outside Moslem and high caste Hindu circles.

ASTEROID BODIES

This unusual type of senile degeneration of the vitreous, characterised by the deposit of calcium soaps as small round bodies, known as asteroids, is found in the older age groups. In the tropics, where old age comes on earlier than in the West, it is a frequent finding, presenting a very striking picture. In a large proportion only one eye is involved. They do not have any sinister significance.

Depending on whether they are viewed by direct illumination or by a beam reflected from the surfaces behind them, the asteroids are white and shiny, spherical or oval, with the appearance of snowballs, or black spots. Sometimes they are spattered with pigment granules. They are generally disseminated throughout the vitreous, but also may be seen in localised clumps. It is noticeable that there may be very little disturbance in the vitreous framework, in other words the vitreous itself has not become fluid. In consequence, the asteroid bodies are suspended in the vitreous and are in no respect mobile, which differentiates them from another condition where crystalline deposits form mobile particles within fluid vitreous (synchesis scintillans). The latter condition occurs in younger individuals with diseased eyes, and is more likely to be bilateral. The particles are larger and brighter than *mf. volvulus*. Asteroid bodies, once seen, cannot be confused with anything else.

THE PROBLEM OF OPTIC ATROPHY

In tropical countries, particularly in those that have been, or are, poor, bilateral optic atrophy poses many diagnostic dilemmas. In West Africa, by the 40th year, optic atrophy is the fourth most common cause of blindness, so the problem it sets is a pressing one. Only by constantly reminding oneself of how optic atrophy develops is it possible to make a diagnosis, and, if it is not too late, commence treatment. *This section takes a lot of reading, but if the headings and italics alone are read, the probable causes should be clear.*

Development of optic atrophy

Vascular occlusion

The optic nerve head is supplied by branches of the posterior ciliary arteries, which are also the arterial source for the posterior uvea, but these are two separate groups of vessels with no connection between their subequent capillary nets (Anderson & Braverman, 1976). These authors have shown in addition that *the optic nerve head capillaries connect with the retinal and retrobulbar (including the pial) microvasculatures.*

These recent findings help to explain some hitherto bewildering clinical observations, as, for example, the obvious nourishment of the disc in the face of marked peripapillary choroidal atrophy. They also explain why *ischaemic optic neuropathy—with initial swelling followed by atrophy of the disc—is more common in the elderly, where presumably it is less likely that these alternative vascular links are efficient;* on the other side of the coin, there is no way of knowing how many subjects, especially the elderly, may not have avoided ischaemic optic atrophy, or have only suffered partial loss, by reason of these same vascular anastomoses.

In middle or old age, *arteritis is one of the commonest reasons* for closure of the nutrient vessels to the optic nerve, with the subsequent development of ischaemic optic neuropathy, and there is no reason to conclude arteritis does not occur in the tropics simply because it has been reported only infrequently, especially as the causes of so many optic atrophies in the tropics remain obscure. *Increased blood viscosity,* as in sickle cell-Hb C, and polycythaemia vera-rubra, may also cause vascular occlusion and lead to an appearance identical to ischaemic optic neuropathy.

In *chronic glaucoma* the mechanism causing ischaemia of the optic nerve head is something different. It seems most likely that rises in intraocular pressure will compress the veins and capillaries, which have weaker walls and lower intravascular pressures, rather than the arteries which have higher pressures and tougher walls; *the haemodynamic pressure in the veins must rise in by far the majority to counterbalance rises in intraocular pressure, or there would be no circulation at all.* It is possible, therefore, to conclude that the blood flow behind the retinal veins is subject to reflex autoregulatory mechanisms in order to maintain a steady flow in the presence of rises and falls of intraocular pressure. *We know that increased resistance to aqueous outflow is the cause of chronic glaucoma.* It is also reasonable to suppose that resistance to raised intraocular pressure based on autoregulatory mechanisms will diminish with time, hence the increase of optic atrophy with age. It takes only one step further to conclude that, *in unresponsive chronic glaucoma with progressive field loss, it is the haemodynamic mechanisms—no longer efficient nor able to resist inconsistent variations of intraocular pressure—which are responsible as much as, if not more than, the defective outflow.* Intermediate phases are bound to be the most confusing.

In *acute glaucoma, optic nerve damage is likely to be purely ischaemic, following compression by the high intraocular pressure of the blood vessels nourishing the optic nerve head.* At first this causes swelling, which resolves after the damage is done, leaving a non-excavated pale optic disc, although a degree of cupping may be present if the original physiological cup happens to be deep. This is true of cupping in all ischaemic optic neuropathies (Douglas et al 1974). Such an appearance, that is a pale, somewhat excavated, but most frequently not deeply excavated, optic cup is quite common in developed countries, but in the writer's experience in the tropics deep cupping is more likely to be present. It is not known whether physiological cups are deeper in the non-Caucasian eye.

Other mechanisms

Mechanisms other than vascular ones also play a part in the production of optic atrophy, *following impairment of the cytoplasmic metabolism, or of the axon cylinders, by poisons* such as lead, quinine, methanol, argemone, etc., *by malnutrition,* usually a deficiency in the B complex, *by metabolic disorders,* such as diabetes, *or by infections* such as cerebrospinal meningitis. These and other similar conditions produ-

cing optic atrophy are all described elsewhere under the appropriate headings.

Details of the main diseases causing optic atrophy now follow.

Glaucoma

In acute glaucoma the optic disc during an attack may be impossible to see due to corneal oedema. The eye is congested, the cornea steamy and the pupil dilated and fixed. Pain is severe and in the tropics, where no treatment is available, this pain remains in the memories of those who have endured it long after it has gone, leaving a clear history and a white, atrophic, deeply cupped optic nerve (Plate 38).

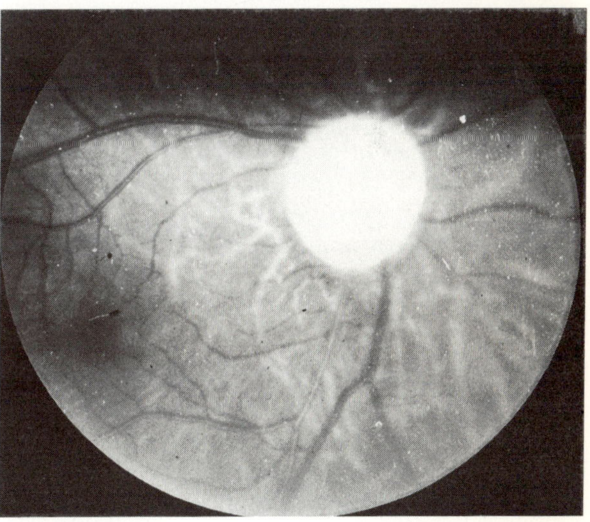

Plate 38 Deep cupping and total optic atrophy in both eyes (in African aged 20) of unknown nature. He was examined fully in England

In chronic simple glaucoma, not infrequently also associated with a short period of severe pain, there is a similar well developed cup, which in the end is associated with a white, atrophic disc. The colour of the disc is accentuated by comparison with the pigmented fundus of those who live in tropical countries. Diagnosis of the glaucomas largely depends on high readings with a tonometer; however, burned-out cases are common and it is not unusual to find a normal tension in the presence of a deep, white, atrophic cup. Plotting the visual fields using the Traquair targets and confrontation is not very reliable, but it is probably more useful than plotting the fields by the techniques of perimetry and scotometry. Glaucoma has been discussed more fully earlier in this chapter.

Argemone poisoning

Argemone oil (Katakar oil in India) is expressed from the seeds of the prickly poppy (Argemone mexicana), which often grows among mustard and so can adulterate mustard oil. The toxic alkaloid in the oil is sanguinarine, which can be isolated.

Poisoning produces epidemic dropsy, which has a variety of physical signs and symptoms, the most striking being oedema of the lower limbs of a solid type. The absence of a peripheral neuropathy distinguishes it from wet beriberi.

Hakim (1954) has elucidated the pharmacological properties of sanguinarine and its action in relation to the intraocular pressure, which rises alarmingly. He has identified the presence of sanguinarine in nearly 50 species of poppy-fumirarias.

This is not a congestive glaucoma despite very high intraocular pressures (70 to 100 mmHg). Cupping appears early and is deep.

Temporal arteritis

The symptoms are well known: malaise, anorexia, weight loss, joint pains, myalgias, headache, usually tenderness of the temporal arteries and sometimes transient loss of vision. Usually the patient is elderly. Where arteritis affects the optic nerve head blood vessels, there will always be some transient, or even permanent, loss of vision, accompanied or followed by swelling of the optic nerve head, a pseudopapilloedema. A greyish white mass has been reported in the nerve fibre layer around the disc. A raised ESR is constant during the acute phase, but pulsation within the temporal arteries can exist despite this, although it may be feeble and affecting one side more than the other. There can be little doubt that *arteritic* anterior ischaemic optic neuropathy is fairly common in developed countries, and only too frequently followed by a high incidence of disc cupping and pallor with loss of sight, although once again the cupping possibly depends largely on the initial size of the physiological cup. It is not known how common, or uncommon, arteritis is in underdeveloped tropical countries, but its existence must be sought.

Toxic neuropathies

These include some of the more common causes of optic atrophy in the tropics. The optic nerve is vulnerable, as has been indicated above, to a wide variety of toxic substances which directly poison the receptors, bipolar and ganglion cells of the retina, one or all, or impair the metabolism of the axon cylinders, or destroy the myelin. In addition to those mentioned on page 67, penicillin and chloramphenicol in excess, *tobacco, certain poisonous glycosides, alcohol,* pentavalent organic arsenicals such as *tryparsamide* (which used to be used overvigorously in the treatment of trypanosomiasis) can all produce hyperaemic swelling of the optic nerve, going on to toxic optic atrophy of a simple type with shallow, but wide, cupping. In all these toxic optic neuropathies there is early interference with conduction within the optic nerve, and so the colour intensity comparison test described in Chapter 1 is helpful in diagnosing functional loss at an early stage. If the colour displayed is less bright in one eye than in the other, then the sign (known as Uhthoff's sign) is said to be positive. Using the large Traquair colour targets it is possible in addition to demonstrate that the red-green targets are not as well seen as the blue-yellow. Retinal lesions do not generally cause red-green defects, although unfortunately blue-yellow defects are sometimes also caused by optic nerve lesions. As these are simple tests, it is worth carrying them out in order to obtain confirmatory evidence of the existence of a toxic neuropathy.

The so-called *tobacco-alcohol amblyopia,* the diagnosis of which depends on the finding of a characteristic centro-caecal depression in the visual fields, no doubt occurs in the tropics, but it is difficult to prove unless the co-operation between the patient and the observer is a good one. There is no fundus pathology to help diagnose this type of toxic neuropathy; moreover the alcohol taken and the quantities of tobacco smoked are always somewhat vaguely described. We are concerned with pipe smoking, and not all who suffer from this condition in the West smoke pipes, but those who do, if they stop smoking a pipe, improve. It is also known that a small minority suffer from *pernicious* (B12) *anaemia* of whom 30 per cent show overt deficiency, and of the latter usually those who suffer from *malabsorption.* The condition recovers with injections of hydroxycobalamine; very few have *folate deficiency,* although these few do respond to treatment with folates. About 30 per cent of tobacco-alcohol cases in the Western World (in addition to the close relationship with B12 deficiency) exhibit *low protein malnutrition*. Further to confuse the issue is the fact that under half are regular drinkers, and generally all these patients are undernourished.

Bronte-Stewart, et al (1976) hold the view that in toxic neuropathy from tobacco-alcohol poisoning there is *a deficiency in sulphur associated with a secondary defect of cyanide metabolism*. Certain sulphur amino acids such as cystine (they claim) are low in the plasma of patients with tobacco-alcohol amblyopia, and when given oral cystine (4 g daily) tobacco-alcohol amblyopia subjects recover vision. *A deficiency of sulphur can occur in protein dietary deficiencies, or where vitamin B12 or folate is deficient in the diet, or as the result of malabsorption.* The role of *pyridoxine* in the elaboration of sulphur amino acids is an important one, and this may be why B complex therapy, which includes pyridoxine, has been reported as helping recovery in tobacco amblyopia. *Sulphur and the B complex are not infrequently deficient in the diets in tropical countries.* With the apparent causative factors all present, more or less, in the remote areas of tropical countries, it is reasonable to think it likely that tobacco-alcohol poisoning should explain many of the toxic optic neuropathies found in such areas; yet it has not been found possible to aid recovery by giving large intramuscular doses either of hydroxycobalamine or of cystine over a period of 6 months to 2 years in sufficient numbers to make the existence of this condition a statistically proven fact, particularly in the absence of reliable visual field plotting.

It has been suggested above that tobacco-alcohol amblyopia is associated with a defect in the cyanide detoxication mechanisms, probably when sulphur amino acids are low in the plasma, and·that hydroxycobalamine facilitates the excretion of hydrocyanic acid (HCN), an effect paralleled by cystine. There is a link here with what is said to occur in the case of several plant foodstuffs in use in the tropics, which contain cyanogenetic glycosides. The quantity of the glycoside depends to some extent on the conditions under which the plant concerned is grown and prepared for food. Bruising or other injury of the foodstuff brings about enzyme action and hydrocyanic acid is set free from the glycoside. *Linamarin is the glycoside of the dolichos and lima bean, sweet potato, gram and manioc (cas-*

sava). The enzyme which frees the contained prussic acid (hydrocyanic acid) is linase. In most of these foodstuffs, all of which, particularly manioc, are staples in large areas of the third world, the glycosides are not likely to give rise to poisoning, either because they are present in very small amounts, or they occur in parts which are not eaten, or because the inhabitants know the risk and prepare the foodstuff accordingly. *In Nigeria all six varieties of cassava grown there contain sufficient amounts of cyanogenetic glycoside to make them toxic.* Most of this lies in the outer coats of the manioc root, and these parts may be easily pealed off. When poisoning occurs it is due to roots (which contain a greater amount of the glycoside than usual) having been badly bruised in the preparation, so that the prussic acid is liberated and spreads throughout the substance. When the roots are boiled, most of the toxic substance is dissolved and removed, but not all. It is important that the cooking pot should not be covered with a lid, so that the volatile HCN can escape with the steam and that the water in which manioc has been boiled is thrown away. The suggestion has been made that when such a contaminated preparation is ingested, or inhaled, this is what poisons the optic nerves. If the amount of prussic acid is gross, then systemic poisoning with giddiness, headache and mental confusion, followed by death, may take place within 2 hours. If the amount is small, but repetitive, the toxic effect on the optic nerves could be cumulative, giving rise to optic atrophy.

The occurrence of primary optic atrophy following the ingestion of the female of the plant *Hagenia abyssinica* in Ethiopia, where it is used to eliminate tapeworms, has already been noted in Chapter 2. Other plant poisons, either accidental or deliberate, may well lead to optic atrophy in some of the more remote regions of the world.

Nutritional amblyopia

The origin of this retrobulbar neuritis, which advances to optic atrophy, is not firmly established, but *all are agreed it is caused by a deficiency of one or more members of the B complex,* and is not a toxic neuropathy. The initial clinical picture resembles any retrobulbar neuritis, namely a period of congestion, perhaps swelling, of the optic discs, and then the gradual onset of pallor, which may affect the temporal part of the optic nerve head only. *Thiamine, riboflavin and nicotinic acid* are primarily involved in the development of beri-beri, the orogenital syndrome and pellagra respectively, yet at some time or another each of these conditions has been reported in association with nutritional amblyopia, and when treated with the B complex retrobulbar neuritis has disappeared. It seems very likely that in certain circumstances a deficiency of any one of these three vitamins affects the function of the optic nerve, although a more complex aetiology is possible. Of the other members of the B group only pyridoxine and *pantothenic acid* should probably be considered. The latter, as well as thiamine, is needed for the oxidation of pyruvate, but the trail ends there; it is seldom deficient.

The majority of nutritional cases which have been examined with care by experts were seen during the second World War in the Middle and Far East. The onset is usually sudden, although apparently there is difficulty in focusing prior to loss of sight. This is the rule in all optic neuropathies. Thus, vision is blurred fairly early at a time when the optic nerves look, and probably are, healthy. Some observers have noted the early onset of oedema and hyperaemia of the discs; others have not observed this, but with the onset of retrobulbar neuritis, a long period of defective vision follows. The only successful treatment on record in the prisoner-of-war camps followed the early administration of intramuscular thiamine (Houwer, 1946). Association with a peripheral neuropathy was common.

Pallor of the discs takes a month or more to develop. The colour intensity comparison test helps to reveal the condition. Cupping is never present unless physiological cups were noted initially. A close relationship between beri-beri and nutritional amblyopia has been noted by Rodger (1952) in British survivors of Japanese prison camps and by King & Passmore (1955) among the American survivors of Korean prison camps. In all these subjects intense physical exertion on high carbohydrate diets lacking the B complex were the rule; these circumstances should be remembered in the tropics; they are not often found, which explains the low prevalence of this condition.

Syphilis

A basal meningovascular *syphilis* at any period of infection commences with severe headaches (especially at night) and papilloedema. Hyperaemia and swelling of the optic nerves may be observed and will advance to atrophy. In addition, cranial nerve palsies occur. If the lesion is focal, a single cranial nerve may be involved, especially a partial third, resulting in a divergent squint. Endemic syphilis, which is more common in the tropics than venereal, is due to contagion from the skin and mucous membranes by the same agent as classic syphilis *(treponema pallidum)*. Because the condition is endemic, it appears that immunity occurs in the majority which, as a rule, prevents the third stage central nervous system lesions developing; this does not, however, exclude the possibility of a basal meningovascular inflammation arising at some stage of the endemic disease, nor of migrants introducing classic strains of venereal syphilis.

Almost certainly serological tests will be unavailable in the areas under consideration. A positive diagnosis by means of a blood WR is not necessarily an indication of syphilitic infection, as biological false positive reactions occur, and a positive blood WR is found in yaws.

The treponema immobilisation test (TPI) and the fluorescent treponemal antibody test (FTA) are more specific and sensitive methods of diagnosis, remaining positive after treatment. A positive serological reaction in blood or c.s.f., or both, would be of particular value in those presenting with an optic atrophy with or without an associated, isolated cranial nerve palsy. *An effort should be made to send some sera in an area where optic atrophy is rife to a central laboratory.*

Onchocerciasis

To quote Bird et al (1976) 'Optic nerve disease alone in the presence of choroidoretinal changes was responsible for a large proportion of blindness due to the posterior segmental lesion in onchocerciasis in the Cameroon (87.6 per cent in this series)'. The author in checking 100 posterior segmental lesion case records in West Africa found 45 per cent had optic atrophy associated. It is interesting to consider what the *modus operandi* may be of onchocercal optic atrophy:

1. Optic neuritis can follow any severe anterior and posterior uveitis. The consequent optic atrophy is

often concealed because of pupillary membranes or secondary complicated cataracts. It arises secondary to destruction of the ganglion cells, or perhaps because the toxin diffuses into the nerve head.

2. A toxic effect on the axon cylinders can occur as a direct effect of the products of the disintegrating bodies of dead microfilariae, which are known to be able to penetrate the optic nerve.

3. Ischaemic optic neuropathy is quite likely following closure of the nutritional blood vessels, or those posterior ciliary arteries supplying the optic nerve head, as a result of toxins liberated around the small vessels by the bodies of dead microfilariae within the nerve head. This effect would reflect exactly what occurs to the capillaries of the skin.

4. The interaction between a dense skin infection (with mf. *volvulus)* and a poor state of malnutrition can precipitate the development of nutritional amblyopia with optic atrophy (Rodger, 1973).

It is known that the greater the density of human infection with onchocerciasis, the greater is the prevalence rate of optic atrophy in such populations. The author believes that all four modes of onset given above occur. In the case of the last-named, it is interesting to note that those presenting with very dense infections, suffering also from malnutrition, had a similar symptomatology to those prisoners of war seen in Japanese and Korean prison camps in 1939 to 1945 mentioned under 'Nutritional amblyopia'.

The subjects exhibit retarded growth, wasting of muscles, a wrinkled, lack-lustre skin, laceration, crusting or fissuring of the outer canthi, nares or outer angles of the mouth, lethargy, uncertain gait and the staring eyes of those who have seriously impaired vision as a result of optic nerve disease. Such patients have been reported to have had all their symptoms cured by the administration of Benerva compound tablets (thiamine hydrochloride 1 mg, riboflavin 1 mg, nicotinamide 15 mg). The result was speedy and dramatic. The sooner treatment is given the better, as there must be some functioning axon cylinders left for there to be any recovery at all. The possibility of a successful response recedes after 6 months.

Among the causes of optic atrophy discussed here, the explanation of any particular one must surely lie. If diagnosed in time, all of them can be prevented.

Other infections

Rare causes include *cerebrospinal meningitis, trypanosomiasis, tuberculosis, relapsing fever, typhus, coccidioidosis, cryptococcosis, paragonimiasis* and perhaps *bilharzia.*

5

Ocular complications of the common tropical diseases

The title 'Ocular complications of the common tropical diseases' is not the same as saying that the ocular complications are common. Sometimes they are (as in measles), sometimes not (as in sickle cell disease). As the systemic diseases are common, the ocular complications must be known, and are described in some detail. The distribution, nature and principal symptoms of the diseases are described (briefly) as an 'aide memoire'. In this way the practitioner is less likely to forget the frequent role systemic diseases play in causing blindness.

CEREBROSPINAL MENINGITIS

The disease and its symptomatology

Cerebrospinal meningitis is endemic throughout the world. It is more frequently seen in epidemic form in the tropics than elsewhere. Twenty-five years ago, throughout West Africa, whole villages were wiped out by epidemics of cerebrospinal meningitis, the few survivors leaving their deserted homes behind as they fled elsewhere. In Delhi in 1966 one third of all infants below the age of 1 died in such an epidemic. Epidemics come in waves, every so many years, and thus it is important when first arriving in a new area to ascertain when the last one occurred.

The organism is a Gram-negative, kidney-shaped, small diplococcus found within and outside the leucocytes in cerebrospinal fluid. There is a greater tendency to variation in size and shape than is the case with gonococcus, which in smears is more uniformly distributed. There appear to be four strains, or groups, of the responsible meningococcus (*Neisseria meningitidis*), none more deadly than another. *Pneumococcus* and *H. influenza meningitis* also occur, especially in West Africa, and *tuberculous*

meningitis, although less frequent, is not unknown.

There are many immune carriers of the organism, but only a few of them ever contract the clinical symptoms; it is the non-carriers who are affected. The prevalence among infants and children is greater than among adults, as the former are less likely to have developed effective immunity. The organisms pass from the nose, mouth and throat of the carrier to the non-immune; excessive dryness of the lining mucous membranes and excessive coughing will in consequence predipose spread. This accounts for the onset of sporadic cases in endemic tropical areas. Epidemics, on the other hand, usually arise during the cold season in the tropics when, at night, the houses and huts are crowded, many of the occupants, including carriers, cough and sneeze, and thus pass the infection on. A decrease in the number of subclinical attacks in the years prior to an epidemic is believed to be another important factor; by reducing the boosting of adequate immunity, the latter becomes inadequate and a seasonal epidemic appears. The conditions described are typical of parts of Africa, Central America, India and Indonesia among other places, occurring in the first two countries mentioned in areas where endemic onchocerciasis exists. There is no problem of diagnosis during an epidemic but the ocular complications of this disease, particularly as far as the uvea is concerned, are hard to categorise in survivors, and in some respects this is also true in the case of the optic nerve.

Diagnosis

Unfortunately, several classic CSM symptoms occur in cerebral malaria (due to *P. falciparum*), in measles, in poliomyelitis and in leptospirosis, in tuberculosis and in several types of virus infection such as Coxsackie, etc. In most of these meningeal irritation (irritability of the patient) is a more important sign than neck stiffness and head retraction.

In isolated cases, examination of the cerebrospinal fluid is clearly an important means of diagnosis. The fluid in lumbar punctures reveals the organisms; in addition it is opaque or purulent (polymorphs), the protein is raised and sugar low. If no organisms are seen and the c.s.f. is clear, a virus is the most likely cause of the meningeal irritation.

One warning word concerns cerebral malaria, the most probable alternative diagnosis to meningitis in tropical countries in isolated cases. As malarial parasites will be present in at least one third of thin blood films examined in any one village (Crewe & Wéry, 1977), it is wise to treat both conditions if in any doubt.

As the standard drugs for meningococcal meningitis are sulphonamides, the effectiveness of which is considerably interfered with by malaria, it is wise to use an alternative, if the condition worsens.

Ocular features

Petechiae on the palpebral, rarely the bulbar, conjunctiva are common early on in about half the patients. An acute endogenous purulent conjunctivitis can be part of a *N. meningitidis* septicaemia; episcleritis is a later manifestation (fifth to sixth day). Exogenous meningococcal conjunctivitis, which may be mild or mucupurulent, has been (rarely) reported in carriers in whom the organism has been isolated from the secretion of the eye as well as from the throat.

There are three serious ocular complications of cerebrospinal meningitis. First, there may be an endogenous anterior uveitis present, sometimes with hypopyon. Inflammatory exudate from the rim of the pupil may occlude it, causing blindness. This membrane is particularly dense and more heavily pigmented after recovery than in any other uveitis, especially in the Negro eye (Plate 39). In some cases endophthalmitis follows uveitis, leading to shrinkage of the eyeball. The second serious complication, leading to blindness in those who survive, is a bilateral optic atrophy. This, no doubt, occurs because in the very young a basal meningitis is common; the simultaneous involvement of the brain stem explains the occurence of various cranial nerve

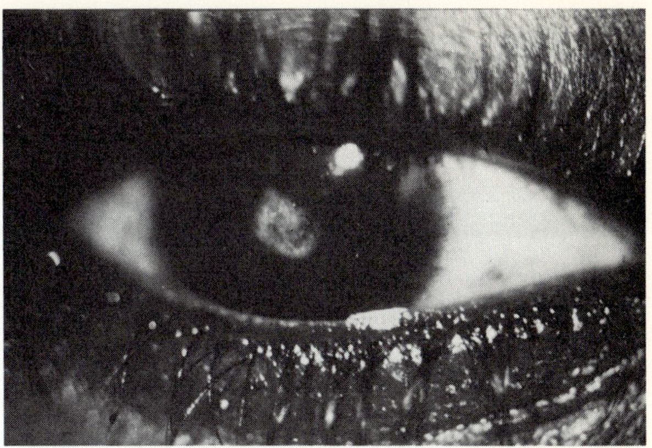

Plate 39 Cerebrospinal meningitis with anterior uveitis. The pupil is covered by a dense pigmented membrane of organised exudate

lesions: a sixth nerve palsy is the most common involvement. Nystagmus is hardly ever noted. The third serious complication is a rarity: it occurs when the meninges in the occipital region are affected; complete blindness with normal fundi and pupillary reactions has been reported. Recovery to hemianopia with return of central vision has been observed in two or three of these cases.

As with any fever, herpes simplex keratitis may complicate the ocular picture.

Treatment

When the anterior uvea becomes involved, good mydriasis is vital, using atropine 1 per cent and phenylephrine 10 per cent 4 hourly. Initial conjunctival injections of 0.10 ml each of mydricaine No. 2 and steroid if available, are also indicated. In addition, topical steroids should be applied four times daily in conjunction with Albucid drops.

For general treatment there are several alternative sulphonamides, which are cheap. Sulphamezathine (sulphadimidine 500 mg) tablets orally, 4 tablets initially and 2 tablets 4 hourly thereafter (with plenty of fluids) is most effective. As an i.m or i.v. injection Sulphamezathine may be given as 1 g in 3 ml of water, the initial injection being one of either 2 or 3g.

Sulphonamide resistance was not reported until 1969, but the resistant strains have only been found in UK and USA, so sulphonamides are still the drugs of choice in the tropics. If the response to them happens to be poor, there are various tetracyclines to choose from.

FILARIASES

The diseases and their symptomatology

Excluding *Onchocerca volvulus* (see Ch. 3), three *Nematode* filarias have been linked with eye changes; they are *Wuchereria bancrofti*, *Brugia malayi* and *Loa loa*; *Dipetalonema perstans* to date has not been implicated. The adult worms survive nearly 20 years in man, the first two in the lymphatics and *Loa loa* in the connective tissue. The microfilariae are all blood-borne and are transmitted as follows:

W. brancrofti Transmitted by:
    Anopheline and Culicine mosquitoes in East and West Africa, South East Asia, South America, Polynesia including Papua New Guinea

B. malayi   Transmitted by:
    Mansonia mosquitoes and some anophelines in Malaya and China.

Loa loa   .Transmitted by:
    Chrysops (mangrove) flies in West and Central Africa, in the Southern Sudan and in the Congo Basin.

The simian Loa is indistinguishable from the human. The presence of any of these three worms is associated with a high degree of eosinophilia.

The symptoms caused by infection with the first two are lymphangitis, abscess formation, arthritis, large groin lymphadenopathy and elephantiasis of the genitalia and legs. *Loa loa* does not produce these complications; it causes itching, sometimes mild, sometimes severe, neuralgias and occasional transient subcutaneous swellings, known as *Calabar swellings*, which probably arise as a result of hypersensitivity, but may arise in an area in which adult worm endotoxin has been excreted excessively. The Calabar swellings are painless and last about 3 days; they never suppurate.

Ocular features

The ocular problems due to loiasis are simple. Apart from Calabar swellings, which may occur by chance on the lids, the adults can appear under the conjunctiva, usually singly, where they can be removed (Plate 40). Because the worm moves fairly quickly, it is wise to paralyse it with a topical anaesthetic and grip it through the conjunctiva with small artery forceps before it disappears. The conjunctiva can then be incised, and the forceps having been removed, the worm is easily withdrawn, provided it is done slowly and gently. It is not known whether mf. loa enters the eye, but it is believed not to. A small intraocular adult *W. bancrofti* (and possibly *B. malayi*) has been definitely identified after recovery from the anterior chamber. If such a parasite were to die there, a severe endophthalmitis would without doubt accrue.

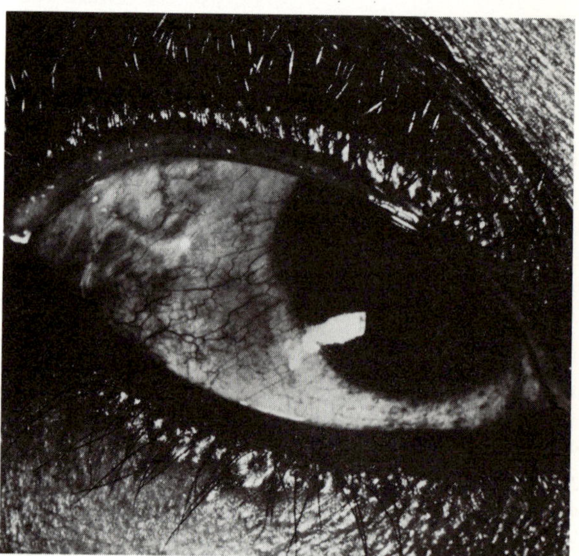

Plate 40 Adult Loa loa under the bulbar conjunctiva

It is now known that the subconjunctival granulomas, known in Uganda as 'Owen Hennessey' granulomas, are almost certainly *Loa loa* of simian origin.

Treatment

Diethylcarbamazine (DEC), about 600 mg a day spread over 3 weeks in divided doses, is an effective treatment against the microfilariae, and if repeated will kill adult Loa loa.

GONORRHOEA AND THE EXTERNAL EYE

Gonorrhoea can affect the uvea and has already been

discussed in this connection on page 45. It is also an important pathogenic organism in relation to diseases of the external eye, which will now be discussed.

The disease and its symptomatology

Neisseria gonorrhoeae (gonococcus) is a Gram-negative, kidney-shaped diplococcus. In smears they are found grouped regularly and extensively in pairs, most lying characteristically within pus or epithelial cells, but some extracellularly. It is the most common and universal of all the venereal diseases, and also spreads by touch transmission.

N. gonorrhoeae is the cause of gonococcal urethritis and vulvo-vaginitis (especially in the young), of gonococcal arthritis, endocarditis, meningitis and septicaemia, and of certain ocular lesions described below.

The natural history of gonorrhoea has changed in the past 50 years; it is less acute now in the West; many patients experience little disturbance and have no complaints. In the tropics, although it still tends to be an acute disease with a profuse urethral discharge, it does not seem to have as severe, nor as many, complications as one would expect.

Gonococci spread directly within the genitourinary tract. Blood-borne complications also occur. In the past gonococcal arthritis associated with a conjunctivitis or a uveitis was said to be common; most cases today are now regarded as being due either to the causative agent of Reiter's syndrome, or to the chlamydial virus which produces non-specific urethral infections. Among ignorant peoples, urine unknowingly infected with gonococci has been used in the past as an eyewash for conjunctivitis with disastrous results.

Ocular features

Gonococcal ophthalmia (neonatorum) is described and discussed in Chapter 3. An exogenous, purulent conjunctivitis occurs in children and adults, arising by touch transmission. It may appear in epidemic form in schools and institutions, and can be associated with an exogenous anterior uveitis. Corneal ulcers also occur with this conjunctivitis, especially when the epithelium is damaged, so great care is required when inserting drops. Such ulcers have been known to perforate the cornea. An endogenous

(blood-borne) granulomatous anterior uveitis is much more common than an exogenous. The most dramatic form it takes is that of a plastic anterior uveitis, with a yellowish gelatinous exudate in the anterior chamber, which causes the pupillary margin to fuse with the anterior lens capsule. Sometimes there is an associated hyphaema or hypopyon. This condition has been well tabulated in the medical literature of the early part of the 20th century, but not very often since. With treatment it clears well.

Treatment

The treatment in cases of penicillin resistance should be by a drug or drop of the tetracycline group. Oral Septrin in adults is most effective after 5 days (2 tablets b.d.) and is not expensive. The paediatric suspension of Septrin is also low priced. Oral therapy should be combined with topical sulphonamide or tetracycline eyedrops or ointment.

MALARIA

The situation today

The epidemiological assessment of the malaria situation is not as hopeful today as it was 10 years ago. More than 1 million people, mainly children, still die from this disease every year, which must surely make it the most serious parasitic disease of all. Repeated resistance of the vectors to adulticides and larvicides and the high cost of drugs continue to block man's efforts to get rid of this debilitating, lethal ailment, and the war to obtain, and then consolidate, eradication is costly beyond the resources of many developing countries. The ocular affections which may be attributed to malaria are few. There are, nevertheless, three important points related to malaria and its treatment affecting the eye which must be mentioned.

Ocular features

Excessive haemolysis

Yellow pigmentation of the conjunctiva is seen in malignant malaria and is not dissimilar to mepacrine staining. The cause is the extensive haemolysis resulting from severe malaria, which is also the reason why retinal haemorrhages are seen from time to time especially in blackwater fever.

Postmalarial herpes simplex

HS keratitis is discussed on page 57. It is believed to be rare in the tropics. However, as an assistant surgeon in Secunderabad after the Second World War, the writer was responsible for 200 beds. During and after the Burma Campaign many Indian soldiers with eye injuries were hospitalised, requiring surgery. The close association of recurrent attacks of malaria in these sepoys, who had been fighting for several years in the Burma Campaign, and the subsequent development of classic dendritic ulcers in the eyes was repeatedly demonstrated. Fortunately, the ulcers appeared to clear up readily with debridement using an orange stick soaked in tincture of iodine. It is impossible to know whether differences in types, or strains, of the malarial parasite or of the herpes simplex virus were responsible for the high incidence of these dendritic ulcers.

Adverse effects of antimalarial drugs

Mepacrine deposits in the bulbar conjunctiva, yellow in colour, have been referred to above. Mepacrine can adopt linear or vortex distribution over the corneal apex, the latter giving rise to the bizarre complaint of blue haloes around lights. Deposition in the cornea is reversible and the retina is not affected.

Chloroquine is another matter. As with mepacrine, deposition of granules, white in colour, occurs in the subepithelium of the cornea. The shape varies from granular lines to fern designs or central vortex dispersion. One eye alone may be affected. White haloes may be the first sign. The corneal changes are reversible. Unfortunately, retinal changes occur which are irreversible, unless caught early. Large daily dosages of 200 to 600 mg Hydroxychloroquine Sulphate prescribed two or three times a day for rheumatoid arthritis, and other collagen diseases, for more than a year can lead to such retinal disasters, which commence either as a foveal pigmentary disturbance, or as a ring of oedema (doughnut effect) around the macula. Central vision is depressed and a central scotoma conforms in shape.

Quinine is still used by many people in the tropics as a prophylactic and, in the presence of resistance to available therapeutic drugs, as a cure. In a small percentage of patients, there is individual hypersensitivity to the drug and sudden blindness in both eyes can occur. Perception of light and the pupillary response can be lost; it may also be associated with permanent deafness. The majority of those affected exhibit a change corresponding to central retinal arterial occlusion (narrow arteries, a white disc and a cherry red spot) with retinal oedema at the posterior pole. Intravenous atropine or Priscol (tolazoline) have been claimed to restore sight, but the author has not found either successful in restoring vision beyond 'finger counting*. Untreated defects in vision due to quinine poisoning may improve by themselves gradually over 6 months. After functional recovery, the arteries appear to remain somewhat narrower than normal and the colour discrimination test reveals a reduction (usually greater in one eye than in the other) of the conduction power of the optic nerves, associated with marked contraction of the fields. Although in experimental animals quinine has been found to poison the ganglion cells of the retina, the exact nature of the lesion in man is not clearly understood. Usually quinine amblyopia occurs in those who have been using quinine as an antimalarial over a long period of time and who, perhaps as a result of a recent severe attack, have increased the dose, but ingestion of large single doses, say as an abortifacient, can also produce sudden loss of vision. Thromboses of the central vessels of both retinas have been recorded as a rarity due to Quinine poisoning.

MEASLES (MORBILLI)

The disease and its symptomatology

In poor communities the world over measles is an important cause of death, especially among small children between 3 months (up to which time they are safe by reason of passive immunity obtained from their mothers) and 3 years. Survivors of an attack are immune for life as a rule. The cause is a highly infective virus, which in all cases not only affects the respiratory tract but also the eye, and indirectly leads to a not inconsiderable amount of impaired vision, unless treated efficiently.

---

*Since going to press the author witnessed a cure from light perception to $\frac{6}{12}$ in a week following injections of 15 ml of 0.5 per cent lignocaine into the stellate ganglia.

Very little epidemiological information on measles is available in South East Asia, where it is known that less than one per cent of the people have been immunised; the case fatality rate despite this appears to be lower than in the old days in Africa before mass measles vaccination programs were introduced. Nevertheless, the disastrous effect of measles, not only in causing death, but also blindness, is still considerable in South East Asia. Meanwhile, the disease in the African continent, where immunisation is being freely practised, has been substantially and quickly brought under control. Ten years ago the mortality rate in Africa was about 20 times greater than in the United Kingdom; now it is only about 2 or 3 times as common.

Diagnosis is difficult in coloured populations, as the distinctive rash, which has to be distinguished from German measles and even scarlet fever, is difficult to see. The classic symptoms in a child suffering from measles consist of nasal and ocular secretions, a harsh cough, often otitis media, and, before the eruption of the rash, the appearance on the anterior portion of the buccal mucous membrane of Koplik's spots, which have the appearance of salt grains on the red mucosa. Anything larger is not likely to be a Koplik spot, but more probably a fungal infection, such as thrush; in the latter the infant may vomit, but is clearly not as seriously ill as is the case in measles. During the period of the spread of Koplik's spots (after the 5th or 6th day) the measly child is fretful, clearly ill and the entire respiratory tract is involved. There is acute photophobia and swelling of the lids. Scarlet fever has to be excluded, but it is not associated with catarrh of the eyes, nose or buccal mucous membrane, as is measles. If the child suffering from measles is seen on the 3rd to 5th day Koplik's spots and the rash may both be present. If seen later, or if the rash arises later, as it sometimes does (for as long as a fortnight after the start of the illness), Koplik's spots will have faded and the only clue is that the buccal mucous membrane is somewhat inflamed and granular. In some instances erosive ulcers of the buccal mucosa in tropical cases advance to produce *Cancrum oris*.

A decrease in the initial acute symptoms coincides with the onset of the rash, which starts behind the ears, spreading downwards. In the pigmented skin, the rash takes the shape of small, irregular, somewhat oedematous patches. As these patches fade desquamation, usually described as being 'like bran', is best

seen over the front of the shoulders when viewed from above and behind.

The most difficult diagnosis to differentiate measles from is that of a severe case of German measles (rubella); in the latter the secretions are usually less and enlargement of the glands quite marked, in particular the occipital glands. Moreover, in German measles desquamation is slight and the palms, both affected in measles, are not affected in rubella at all.

Ocular features

During the acute fever, when the eyes are watering and there is marked photophobia, widely dispersed, *epithelial punctate corneal opacities* arise. These opacities are small and have been recorded as lasting up to 13 weeks after the illness has passed (Florman & Agatston, 1962). They usually disappear without trace in the end.

With fluorescein staining, which helps demonstrate the corneal changes as readily as Rose Bengal, the superficial punctate keratitis is seen to be associated with multiple erosions, not only in the cornea, but on the bulbar conjunctiva of both eyes as well. Early on the lesions cover the entire cornea, but when seen later, they are more commonly present in the area of the palpebral fissure, which is the last to clear. The preauricular glands are not enlarged or tender, except perhaps during the time of Koplik's spots. This keratoconjunctivitis of measles is not associated with follicular or papillary hypertrophy, although in the very early stages the congestion of the palpebral conjunctiva is such that it is difficult to see. The secretion, initially watery, becomes mucopurulent as *secondary bacterial infections* intervene. As a result of these infections *corneal ulceration* (characteristically at the apex) with or without perforation may develop. A dense white leucoma remains if the child survives. If perforation occurs, endophthalmitis and phthisis bulbi may result; alternatively, if the eye heals, the iris is usually seen impacted in the white scar. This condition is known as *leucoma adherens*. This appearance is invariably bilateral, but can be unilateral, and is very suggestive of measles when seen in a blind child (Plate 3).

An associated detrimental factor when a child is suffering from measles with involvement of the corneas is xerophthalmia, which can go on to keratomalacia, because all the factors which produce the latter exist. In the tropics, when a child runs a high temperature, as in measles, the mother invariably takes it outside into the cool air to catch the evening breeze and bathes its head and body with cold water to cool the fever. The result is it catches a chill, with the onset of pneumonia, which gives rise to an added demand for protein and vitamin A, already deficient in the weanling child. It is not to be wondered at in the circumstances that xerophthalmia and keratomalacia so frequently complicate measles. These sick children are at the onset deficient in protein and vitamin A, for, as weanlings they have no passive immunity left and the substitute diet, as has been described in Chapter 3, is inadequate. The watery diarrhoea consequent upon the lack of protein leads to decreased absorption of whatever vitamin A or provitamin may exist in the diet and so the presence of measles puts the sight at great risk. If that were not enough, herpes simplex keratitis may also be associated with measles. As measles is common in hyperendemic trachoma areas, this is another factor which makes the onset of blindness not at all surprising.

A secondary retinitis pigmentosa caused by the morbilli virus is described in Chapter 4 (p. 64).

Treatment

Village health instructions about correct nursing, about cleansing the external eyes and about giving dietary supplements are extremely important. The ideal scheme during an outbreak of measles should include segregation of non-infected children, boosting the diet in all of them, whether they suffer from measles or not (as by giving cod liver oil and soya bean gruel) and the administration of a prophylactic bactericidal by mouth. Treatment of the eyes of children with acute measles is largely symptomatic; a mydriatic and antibiotic drops should be inserted three times a day.

SICKLE CELL DISEASES

The diseases and their symptomatology

The term 'sickle cell disease' is applied to all hereditary disorders in which the red cells contain haemoglobin-S, designated Hb-S; normal haemoglobin is designated Hb-A. Sickle cell disease is inherited as a mendelian dominant; it occurs in Negroes or in those with mixed Negro blood. About 9 per cent of the Negro population in the USA carry Hb-S. In Africa the figure is much higher; it may be as high as 25 per cent.

In the heterozygote, where one Hb-S gene is inherited from one parent and one Hb-A from the other, the cells do not contain sufficient Hb-S for them to undergo sickling even at the lowest oxygen tensions, but such a subject is said to possess the *sickle cell trait* (AS); the red cells in a stained film are normal apart from the presence of about 4 per cent of Mexican hat or target cells. There is good evidence to suggest that to possess the sickle cell trait confers a relative resistance to *P. falciparum* malaria, so that in areas of malarial endemicity the mortality rate is less and this is a factor in the persistence and high frequency of the Hb-S gene in Africa.

When a subject inherits one Hb-S gene from each parent, the resultant homozygous state, designated as sickle cell disease (SS) is sufficient to cause the phenomenon known as sickling to occur in all the offspring (about 1 per cent of all Negroes in the USA). Sickling describes the sickle or crescent shape which red cells adopt where the oxygen tension is reduced most *in vivo,* that is in the small arterioles, the capillaries and the small venules. Haemoglobin types are many and various, but only one associated with the sickle cell trait causes ocular disease, and that is when one parent has a Hb-S gene and the other a Hb-C gene (sickle cell Hb-C disease or SC). The anaemia characteristic of sickle cell disease (SS) may be more severe than in sickle cell Hb-C disease, but for some reason that is not clearly understood the ocular changes are less severe. They are described below.

In the double heterozygous state for Hb-S and thalassaemia genes, rare in Negroes unless their blood is mixed with Mediterranean peoples, the ocular changes are least severe of all. In thalassaemia there is a decreased rate of synthesis of the fetal haemoglobin to adult haemoglobin. Sickle cell thalassaemia (STh) cannot be definitely distinguished from sickle cell disease (SS) by electrophoresis since the two disorders can produce identical patterns, but family studies usually enable a diagnosis to be made.

To sum up, the sickle cell diseases which cause ocular disease in Negro races consist of the double sickle cell gene (often simply called sickle cell anaemia), sickle cell Hb-C disease and to a slighter extent sickle cell thalassaemia disease.

Ocular features

Classically, small thromboses occur in the periphery of the retina at the equatorial-junction zone, where the smallest capillaries exist. While these early changes, with or without associated haemorrhages, may regress in sickle cell anaemia, leaving a scar with a pigmentary reaction, their presence in sickle cell Hb-C disease, in which they are twice as common, is much more likely to be persistent.

These changes stem from increased viscosity, as sickling occurs in capillaries, arterioles and venules with increasingly low oxygen tensions. The circulation becomes slowed and small groups of sickle cells become impacted in various parts of the vessels, which appear to collapse on either side. Small plugs of this nature can be seen in the conjunctival vessels as well as in the fundus. They have recently been noted on the optic nerve head, the appearance being one of small, dark red, round spots. There is no doubt that this is a helpful sign in an African (in whom diabetes is less likely). These red spots do not always remain, but may clear; on the other hand, they can enlarge and lead to vascular blockages with haemorrhages around the optic nerve head (in about 5 per cent of cases).

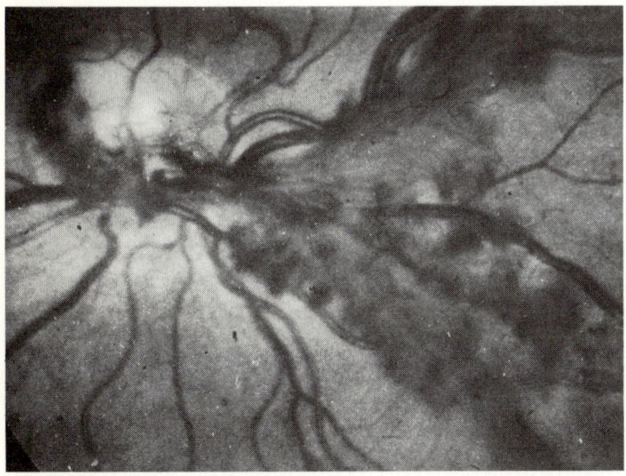

Plate 41 A cluster of new vessels in diabetic retinopathy, not to be confused with the 'sea fan' of sickle cell disease

The most striking changes follow neovascularisation; the anoxia of retinal vascular occlusion leads to the formation of an elaborate network of convoluted interanastomosing vessels, with some arteriovenous fistulas. They occur within the retina in the first instance, although they may eventually break out into the vitreous. The new vessels, attempting to compensate for the lack of oxygen, lie in a delicate matrix of mesenchymal cells, from which vascular endothelial elements and fibrous tissue arise. Such structures are called 'sea fans' (Plate 41). When the 'sea fan' grows into the vitreous, it moves slowly with the movement of the vitreous, hence the use of that descriptive term. The vessels within the 'sea fan' may leak into the matrix, ultimately to grow into the retina, or through the retina into the vitreous, a condition known as 'proliferating retinopathy'. As a rule, however, the fibrous tissue element in the 'sea fan' sooner or later becomes more dense and outweighs the vascular element, so that the new vessels regress as a result of the increased fibrosis; the condition is then called 'retinitis proliferans'.

The developments associated with the formation of a 'sea fan' are more common in the peripheral retina and at the optic nerve head than in the central retina. They can appear in more than one site. Attachment of proliferating fibroblasts, whether in the vitreous or not, from one part of the retina to another may possibly lead to the development of holes or secondary detachments. However, healing and regression of a proliferating retinopathy, even when there is leakage into the vitreous, can occur without leaving anything other than a pigmented scar; this happens in about half of them. In sickle cell Hb-C disease about 5 per cent exhibit in addition angioid streaks, although in no instance has the macula been reported damaged by the latter.

The complications of peripheral sickle cell retinopathy have been assessed as follows:

Vitreous haemorrhages	6 to 7 per cent
Retinal traction bands (with or without detachment	1 to 5 per cent
Blindness in one eye	10 to 20 per cent

As diabetic and hypertensive retinopathies are being increasingly reported from Africa, the recognition of sickle cell changes is vital.

Treatment

There is no ocular treatment for these changes. Photocoagulation is used where available to burn up new tissue and seal leaking vessels, but the results are invariably disappointing.

TREPONEMATOSES (the syphilides)

Syphilis (like tuberculosis) poses problems in all countries of the world. Both these diseases affect the eye in a multitude of ways, the lesions being frequently difficult to distinguish from each other. The ophthalmologist from the Western World often knows far less about syphilis and tuberculosis and their ocular complications than his counterpart in developing countries, because the numbers affected in developed countries have been greatly diminished since the introduction of specific drugs, which cure both conditions.

The diseases and their symptomatology

The origin of the treponematoses has been comprehensively described by Wilcocks & Manson-Bahr (1972). Clinically and epidemiologically there are differences between the diseases caused by the different spirochaetes: the *Treponema pallidum* of venereal and endemic (non-venereal) syphilis, the *Treponema pertenue* of yaws and the *Treponema carateum* of pinta—although they may be varieties of the same strain. These treponemes are morphologically identical, and serological tests have failed to differentiate them.

Yaws (framboesia)

The disease is found in the Caribbean, South America, Africa, the Far East, and even in North Australia. Transmission is by direct contact from the papules. The primary lesion is a granular papilloma, usually ulcerated and healing by scab formation. The secondary stage consists of aches and pains, a fever and crops of papules, some oozing but usually dry, distributed throughout the body, even on the soles of the feet. These papules do not contain true granulation tissue. In the tertiary stage, ulcers and necrotic granulomas (gummas) occur. Healing is by scarring. Evidence of the latter must be sought in late cases in order to make a diagnosis. A chronic ulcerating lesion can affect the nose, or orbit, giving rise to destruction of underlying bone and cartilage with tissue loss (gangosa).

Bone lesions are common in the secondary stage; the tibia is not infrequently thickened and bowed (sabre tibia) as are the hand bones and ulnas, as in venereal syphilis.

In tertiary yaws the gummata, which leave characteristic thin depigmented scars after healing, involve the bones and joints less frequently than occurs in the secondary stage, but also give rise to severe bone pain, swellings and deformities due to new bone formation. On scar tissue being formed, contractures of joints and crippling deformities, especially of the bony extremities, occur. As in *endemic* syphilis, the eye in yaws, and the cardiovascular and central nervous systems escape damage.

Mass campaigns with penicillin have greatly reduced rural yaws, but men cured of yaws who visit cities or ports can contract venereal syphilis, and on returning home in the secondary phase can infect their children directly via the skin with venereal syphilis. This may confuse the diagnostician unless he asks whether people have travelled and to where.

Healing of the face by scarring gives rise to deformities including ectropion of the lower lids. This and destruction of an eye and orbit in *yaws gangosa* are the only ocular lesions found.

Pinta

Pinta is endemic in the Americas from Mexico to Cuba. It differs somewhat from African yaws. The skin lesions consist of dry and scaly papules which are irritable. Scratching leads to oozing, and as the secretion contains *T. carateum* this leads to transmission by contact; so it is yet another 'crowded house' disease. In the tertiary stage depigmentation occurs with coloured or grey patches of various sizes. Pruritus is marked during the acute secondary stage and is still present during the tertiary to a greater or lesser degree. Primary lesions involving the lids may produce scarring and deformities.

Non-venereal syphilis

This manifestation of syphilis is endemic north of the equator in Africa and in Western and Central Asia. It is transmitted by contagion from infectious lesions of the skin and mucous membranes. Venereal transmission is uncommon, but not impossible. Primary and secondary stage lesions similar to yaws and to venereal syphilis occur, but the eye, the cardiovascular system and the central nervous system are only rarely affected. There seems little doubt that the existence of so many areas of endemic non-venereal syphilis in the tropics explains why the ocular manifestations are less common than they used to be in the Old World.

Venereal syphilis

In the primary stage there is a single (usually) sore or 'chancre', which can be found on the genitalia, lip, nipple, anus or finger. It becomes an indurated, painless ulcer, discharging serum which contains *T. pallidum.* In the secondary stage, associated with the systemic spread of the organism, there is a mild illness, a sore throat and a polymorphic eruption of small papules (initially macules), the lack or irritation of which is characteristic. It may become secondarily infected. *A special feature is the recurrence of similar secondary stage mucocutaneous lesions after a period of quiescence.*

Tertiary, or late, syphilis affects the skin, eye, cardiovascular system and central nervous system. The essential lesion in all areas is the formation of granulation tissue. When circumscribed (best seen in the skin) the lesion is called a 'gumma'; gummata are circumscribed, necrotic, infective lesions.

The commonest sites, apart from the skin, are the aorta or other large vessels, the eye, or the meninges and base of the brain. The ocular lesions are described later under ocular features.

Congenital syphilis

Infection by placental transfer (about the 16th week onwards) occurs generally during the later months of pregnancy. Signs of infection may be almost immediate. The child often presents with a secondary syphilitic rash, having failed to thrive. Ulceration occurs around the mouth and nose, eroding the cartilage. Hepatomegaly, splenomegaly and widespread periosteitis, which causes new bone formation and double contour (in consequence) to the shafts, usually of long bones, also occur. Permanent dentition is defective. Thus, the triad of lesions typical of congenital syphilis are all there: 'saddle' nose, 'sabre' tibia and 'Hutchinson's' teeth. Involvement of the cardiovascular system and central nervous system are seen at birth or soon afterwards. Clinical manifestations of meningitis are less common than in the juvenile.

The simpler serum tests likely to be available cannot distinguish syphilis from yaws. In certain acute conditions, for example glandular fever and virus pneumonia, these tests may also be transiently positive. In a few chronic infections a weak and consistently positive WR test may be found, as in malaria and leprosy. Thus the diagnosis is made very much on the strength of the history and physical findings.

Primary luetic lesions in patients are cutaneous, local and associated with enlargement of the lymph nodes. The secondary lesions are bloodborne and more widespread, depending on inflammatory exudation, but can resolve with little or no fibrosis. In the tertiary stage, granulation tissue forms in association with an arteritis, which causes ischaemic necrosis. Spontaneous healing by replacement fibrosis is slow. In the case of the cornea, the symptomatology and course is much altered by the development of tissue hypersensitivity to the invading pathogen, but primary granulation around spirochaetes also plays a part. It seems probable that in the case of the uvea the same mechanism is involved, as Foerster (1959) demonstrated.

Ocular features

Involvement of the eye is found in congenital or acquired venereal syphilis; there is some doubt if it occurs in endemic syphilis unless cases of venereal syphilis co-exist in the endemic areas. Every structure of the eye is affected. Syphilis is still classed as one of the important causes of both anterior and posterior uveitis. The corneal change known as interstitial keratitis is classic within the first year of a primary infection. A basal meningovascular syphilis, if untreated, can give rise to squints (affecting the sixth, or part of the third nerve), pupillary anomalies, ptosis, deafness and facial palsy. Neuroretinitis and optic atrophy also occur and can cause blindness. As said earlier, you cannot leave syphilis out of the reckoning as the cause of any ocular lesion in an area where venereal syphilis exists. The lesions now to be described are those most likely to be seen in Afro-Asia or the Arab World, whether in a small hospital or when visiting villages.

Interstitial keratitis

This is the classic ocular finding of congenital syphilis, occurring in about 10 to 15 per cent of cases. It also occurs in acquired syphilis. Interstitial keratitis (IK) appears between the ages of 2 and 20, may be

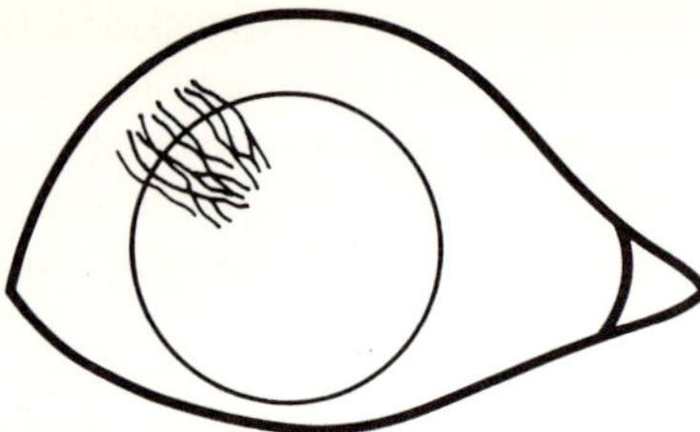

Fig. 5.1 A 'salmon patch' in active syphilitic interstitial keratitis. The localised group of intracorneal vessels is full of blood, hence the name

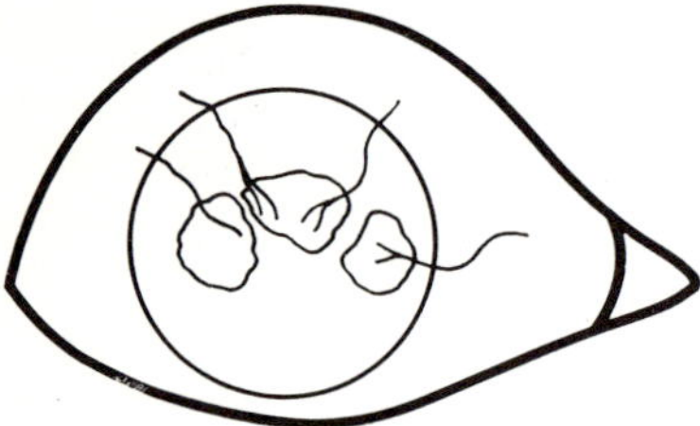

Fig. 5.2 Old scars and interstitial (stromal) vessels in quiescent or healed syphilitic interstitial keratitis. The vessels being empty of blood are thin and grey in colour (ghost vessels)

unilateral at first, but usually becomes bilateral, and is associated with lacrimation, photophobia and pain. There is a quickly increasing corneal haze, as infiltration and new vessel formation increase, particularly in the posterior half of the corneal stroma. In 95 per cent of cases IK is associated with a mild anterior uveitis. The deep new vessels are usually most profuse in one sector of the eye, giving rise to a dull, reddish pink colour in that situation, known as a 'salmon patch' (Fig. 5.1). The eye is congested and the uveitis may involve the anterior choroid as well as the iris and ciliary body. The condition is self-healing, becoming chronic; it is not destructive, but leaves behind large, grey, polyhedral corneal subepithelial patches, with empty blood vessels (ghost vessels) in their neighbourhood. There is nothing which resembles this apart from the interstitial keratitis of tuberculosis and (perhaps) trypanosomiasis. Deep corneal scars (nebulae) and ghost vessels are diagnostic signs of congenital lues, and persist throughout life (Fig. 5.2). The process may remain active for 1 week or several years, and the final result, as far as vision is concerned, also varies considerably.

Congenital syphilitic chorioretinal changes

Scattered patches of chorioretinal atrophy, generally peripheral, occur and may be associated in congenital syphilis with interstitial keratitis. The scars consist of black spots, surrounded by a yellowish-white circle. These changes are nearly always binocular. One rarely sees the active lesion. The feature, however, most characteristic of congenital syphilis is the 'pepper and salt' fundus, where all but the posterior pole of the fundus is covered with minute bluish-black dots, between which lie equally minute dots of depigmented retina. These changes are accentuated the further out one looks in the fundus. They occur in the retinal pigment epithelium. A pseudo-retinitis pigmentosa may also be seen in a congenital syphilitic eye as a rarity. This is discussed in the previous chapter.

Anterior uveitis

An anterior uveitis largely affecting the iris is said to be by far the most important ocular disease of early syphilis. Woods (1961) says that in the Americas it occurs in approximately 4 per cent of all cases of acquired syphilis. A generalised granulomatous anterior uveitis, this same author also states, occurs in from 1 to 3 per cent of patients with late tertiary syphilis. The early condition is sometimes characterised by the presence on the iris face of small 'varicose' capillary bundles, visible to the naked eye, dotted here and there over the face of the iris in small discrete nests (iritis roseata). Later they increase in size to become papules (iritis papulosa) and later still become large enough to be defined as nodules (iritis nodosa). Otherwise the appearances are those of a classic granulomatous iritis. In the Negro eye aggregation of melanophores conceals these lesions to a great extent.

Disseminated chorioretinitis

This is the most common manifestation of acquired syphilis (Plate 42). It appears particularly in the late secondary stages of the disease, but its onset may be delayed for 10 or more years after infection. In about half the cases it is unilateral. Starting in the usual way with an exudation into both the retina and vitreous, so that vision is reduced and areas of acute inflammation can just be seen in the fundus; the inflammatory foci, few or numerous, in the end heal, adopting small polymorphic shapes, heavily pigmented. That is the usual, but not the only, picture. As a rule the

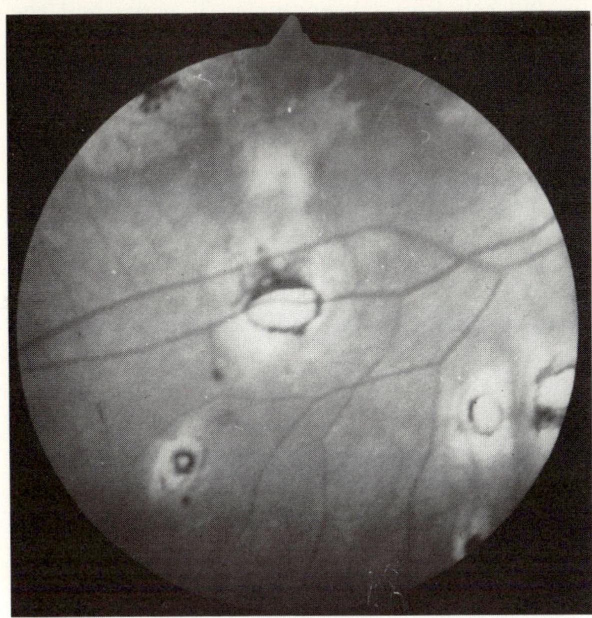

Plate 42 Disseminated chorioretinitis in congenital syphilis

posterior segment of the fundus is preferentially affected, especially for some reason, around the optic nerve head. The retinal vessels are involved in the inflammatory process; there may be exudates and superficial haemorrhages or white vascular sheathing, indicating an arteritis or periarteritis. When the condition heals, occasionally the more peripheral of these vessels may be covered here and there with pigment, forming corpuscular cuffs and aggregations, resembling not only primary retinitis pigmentosa (common in Asia but less common in Africa), but also found in the posterior degenerative lesion of onchocerciasis (see p. 64). In syphilis these pigmentary changes, when they occur, tend to be far more dense and widespread than in either of the other two conditions, and in the Negro eye particularly the whole fundus may be splashed with black patches of pigment dovetailing with white chorioretinal scars.

Treatment

Therapy consists in treating the systemic disease with penicillin or erythromycin, and the ocular lesions with cycloplegics and, if available, topical steroids. Intramuscular penicillin (250 000 units 6-hourly) is given for 10 days. Erythromycin is given in doses of 1 to 2 g daily also for 10 days as may oral Penicillin-V.

TRYPANOSOMIASIS (sleeping sickness)

African trypanosomiasis

The disease and its symptomatology

This is a disease of rural people, exposed to frequent biting by the tsetse fly (*Glossina*). The parasite is a haemoflagellate living in the tissues of its host. At least 35 million people are at risk. There are some areas infested with tsetse for years that have for some reason escaped invasion by the parasite. In endemic areas only about 0.1 per cent of the flies are infected. There are two forms of the disease: the chronic type of disease (which has a short, febrile phase), is caused by a protozoan called *Trypanosoma brucei gambiense*, and is found in West, East and Central Africa. It has a man-fly-man cycle. The flies breed along the rivers—frequently alongside the flies which are the vectors of river blindness. Here the ground is fertile and the population relatively dense and there is excellent bush in which the flies can rest and breed. The incidence rate keeps rising steadily until, or unless, control is instituted. The second, acute, type of the disease is caused by *Trypanosoma brucei rhodesiense* and is found in East Africa. In this case, there is an animal–fly–man transmission in addition to a man–fly–man cycle. The animals concerned are generally cattle and antelope. *T. br. rhodesiense* is by choice a parasite of wild game, less adapted to man than to animals, although it bites man. In consequence, infection with *T. br. rhodesiense* is a chance occurrence over large areas where game and tsetse co-exist, the very areas where usually there is no medical aid of any kind. A third trypanosome (*T. br. brucei*) is infective to animals only.

The site of the bite is relatively painless, although it may develop into quite a large boil. About 3 weeks later trypanosomes appear in the peripheral blood, having arrived there through the lymphatics and lymph glands; enlarged cervical glands are a very important clinical sign. Finally, the parasites enter the cerebrospinal fluid. As a result of the general dissemination within the blood, systemic symptoms occur, with fever, listlessnes and (sometimes) erythema. The terminal stage, the result of a chronic meningoencephalitis, leads to coma and death. Infections with *T. br. gambiense* run a more chronic course than those with *T. br. rhodesiense*, and are less quickly fatal, but the infections are in essence identical.

Ocular features

There is in some patients slight photophobia with congestion of the eyes associated with a diffuse stromal corneal opacification (interstitial keratitis); new vessels grow deeply into the cornea. The condition responds well to specific treatment, unlike syphilitic and tubercular interstitial keratitis, which are known to be hypersensitivity lesions.

This assumes that it is the presence of the trypanosomes in the cornea which is entirely to blame for the interstitial keratitis. The success of therapy in clearing the interstitial keratitis is strong evidence, but trypanosomes are known to elicit in addition an antibody response elsewhere. The interstitial keratitis of sleeping sickness requires to be differentiated from onchocercal stromal keratitis, as both diseases occur in the same regions; in the latter there is always a superficial sclerosing keratitis associated with the interstitial stromal changes, and that is the main differentiating factor.

An anterior uveitis may be seen, perhaps affecting only one eye, with or without corneal involvement. It is granulomatous or mixed in type and may be associated with a hyphaema. It is invariably combined with a tell-tale swelling of the outer part of the lower lids. An antibody response explains the lid swelling and the nongranulomatous part of the mixed anterior uveitis.

In the terminal stages papilloedema, ophthalmoplegias, papillitis and optic neuritis have been reported, especially in *T.br.rhodesiense* infections.

Treatment

Three drugs have been used to treat African sleeping sickness: suramin, pentamidine and (when the central nervous system is involved) melarsoprol. All are dangerous. The danger of tryparsamide (and Atoxyl) has already been mentioned in 'The problem of optic atrophy' (Ch. 4).

American trypanosomiasis (Chagas' disease)

The disease and its symptomatology

Chaga's disease varies from African trypanosomiasis

by the causative trypanosome, *T. cruzi* and the vectors, which consist of some 26 species of the blood-sucking (triatomide) reduviid bugs, either in the larval, nymphal or adult stage. The adult bug can fly considerable distances and voids the trypanosomes when feeding on man. *T. cruzi,* present in the adult bug's excreta, then gain entrance to the host through the insect bite. At least 10 million people have been infected in this way. Chagas' disease is a systemic, often chronic disease. The sore produced by the initial bite is called a 'chagoma'. Systemic spread is quicker than in African trypanosomiasis (only 5 days). Even as *T. br. rhodesiense* may have an animal-fly-man cycle, so does Chagas' disease; among the animals involved may be a dog, rat, bat or cat.

Ocular features

A chagoma sometimes occurs near the eye, and the reduviid bug preferentially bites the face (hence the term 'kissing bug'). In these cases a red, oedematous swelling of the tissue around the eye (Plate 43)

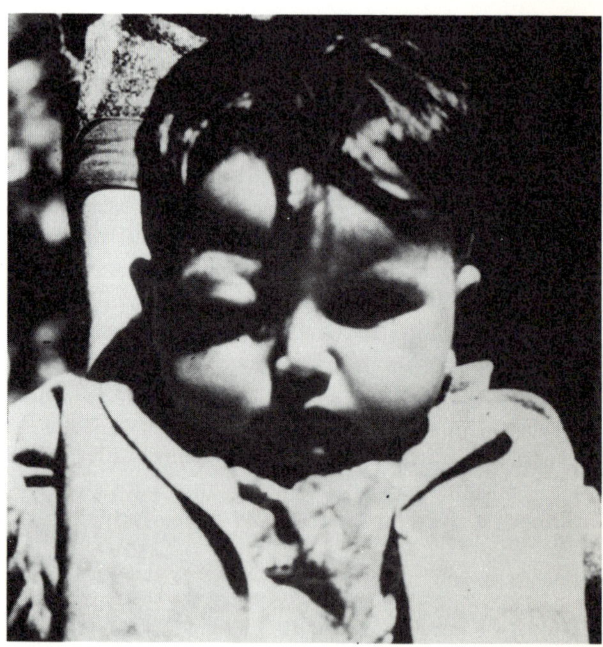

Plate 43 Romana's sign (unilateral palpebral oedema) in Chagas' disease

arises, which causes the lids to close. A chagoma may involve the lacrimal sac (Plate 44). No proven intraocular lesion has been described as yet in an

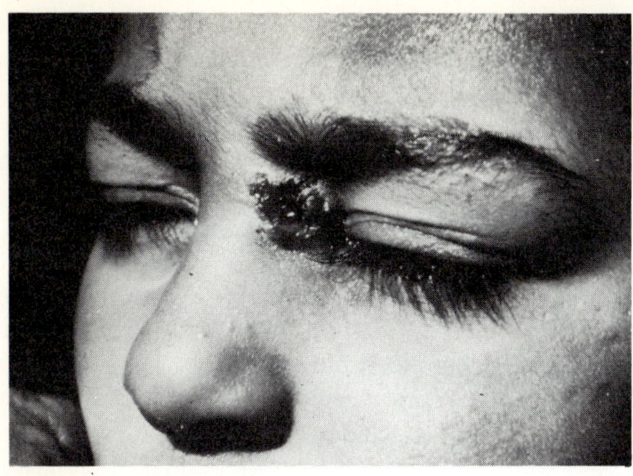

Plate 44 A chagoma involving the lacrimal sac in American trypanosomiasis

acquired case. Atias and his colleagues (1963) in a prematurely born baby (who died 17 days after birth) reported the presence of a granulomatous uveitis. At post-mortem a lymphocytic infiltration of the uvea and retina was found, and *T. cruzi* were present in the infiltrate. No adult case have been confirmed.

Treatment

Until recently no drug was available for the treatment of Chagas' disease. Two compounds, nifurtimox and a derivative of nitro-imidizole have recently been introduced, but are still under trial.

TUBERCULOSIS

The disease and its symptomatology

The dramatic fall in the prevalence of tuberculosis as a disease in developed countries has distracted attention from the magnitude of the tuberculosis problem in developing countries. In most parts of Africa, India, Pakistan, Sudan, the Fertile Crescent, South East Asia, Central and South America it is rife. It is estimated from sputum smear samples that perhaps 15 million cases of *pulmonary* tuberculosis exist in the tropics; the figure for abdominal tuberculosis is not known. Measles, kwashiorkor and gastroenteritis precipitate infection by tuberculosis by lowering the resistance and allowing the tubercle bacilli to gain a

foothold. The reverse is also true. Resistance is of two types: natural resistance present at birth and acquired, due to the development of immunity from a previous infection. Tuberculin reactions indicate past or present infections (see Ch. 7). They have limited diagnostic value.

The only indication of primary tuberculosis in the child may be one of two hypersensitivity states, which represent an allergic reaction to infection, not only with the tubercle bacillus but other bacteria as well, namely erythema nodosum and phylctenulosis. They usually occur after the second year of life, most commonly between the ages of 5 and 20 in the tropics. An uncomplicated primary infection otherwise usually passes unnoticed where X-ray facilities do not exist.

The causative bacillus is *Mycobacterium tuberculosis,* an acid-fast bacillus. This group of rod-shaped bacteria also includes the leprosy bacillus. The technique of staining is given in Chapter 7.

Extension within the lung may occur by recurrent haematogenous spread, but more commonly after a pre-existing focus has eroded a bronchus, by bronchogenous dissemination.

Duke-Elder & Perkins (1966) referring to the extraordinary pleomorphism of the lesions in the eye in tuberculosis aptly state that the controversy surrounding these manifestations results from 'variations in the virulence and massiveness of the infection, and the degree and nature of the resistance put up by the host, depending on his state of immunity and allergy. More frequently the inflammatory reaction incited is nondescript in character and shows nothing in its clinical picture indicative of its pathology'. From such nondescript pleomorphism, personal clinical bias enters into any diagnosis of ocular tuberculosis.

Before the last war tuberculosis was blamed for nearly every obscure ocular lesion, many of which are now clearly non-tubercular, such as toxoplasmosis. Nevertheless, in developing countries where open tuberculosis is common, ocular lesions must be considered likely. In the absence of diagnostic methods of serology and radiology, it is only possible to make a tentative diagnosis by sputum smear. If we exclude the forms in which it is clinically impossible to make a definite diagnosis, one is nevertheless left with a few characteristic ocular changes, which will now be described.

Ocular features

Phlyctenulosis (phlyctenular keratoconjunctivitis)

This disease is not just the result of sensitisation to the human tubercle bacillus, but to other bacilli, although tubercle is the most usual cause in the tropics. It is discussed under the section headed 'Other forms of conjunctivitis' in Chapter 3. The incidence seems to be much greater in Asia than in Africa.

Conjunctival tuberculomas

Primary tuberculosis of the eye and its adnexa is rare, but tuberculomas of the conjunctiva have been reported. Nodular or oozing they are associated with intractable conjunctivitis (Plate 45).

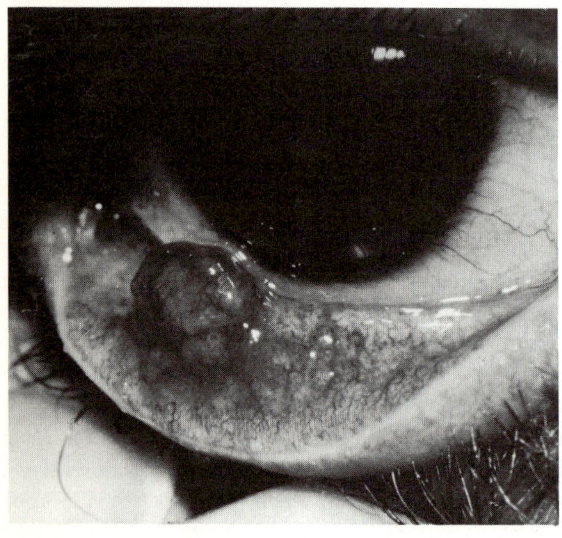

Plate 45 Tuberculoma in lower fornix

Interstitial keratitis

An interstitial keratitis identical to that seen in congenital syphilis, and described under the head, is also caused by tuberculosis.

Tuberculomas of inner eye

Single or multiple tuberculomata are not only found on the surface of the conjunctiva but within the eye on the iris face. In the iris the nodules (tubercles) are multiple and small (miliary) without any surrounding inflammatory reaction. However, if the tissues become hypersensitive, acute inflammation and larger tubercles may be seen. Somewhat similar to the miliary tubercles of the iris are miliary tubercles of the choroid, which complicate the end stages of a fatal tuberculous meningitis in children, as they are the result of a terminal bacillaemia; there is an absence of any inflammatory reaction. The so-called 'solitary' tubercle of the choroid is not common, but it has been noted recently in children in Asia. There is an early active stage, frequently associated with a haemorrhage around a well-outlined solid nodule, and later an exudate may arise, which partially or completely obscures the outline of the solitary tubercle. In the final stage the haemorrhage and exudate are absorbed; the central tubercle becomes either hyalinised or calcified; the end picture is a smooth yellowish-white circumscribed mass, occupying perhaps one-third of the fundus, rather similar to disciform degeneration of the macula.

Granulomatous uveitis

This ocular lesion, classically attributed to tuberculosis, has nothing specific to it. It is rare in patients with active pulmonary disease. In India it is more commonly associated in young people with *abdominal* tuberculosis. In the Americas, some of these eyes have been shown to contain nematodes or *Toxoplasma gondii*. It seems certain that tuberculosis is not as important a cause of chronic granulomatous uveitis as previously claimed. The classic appearance, nevertheless, is well worth noting. There are characteristic yellow, grey or white deposits on the posterior surface of the cornea (mutton fat or lardaceous KP); with the biomicroscope efflores-

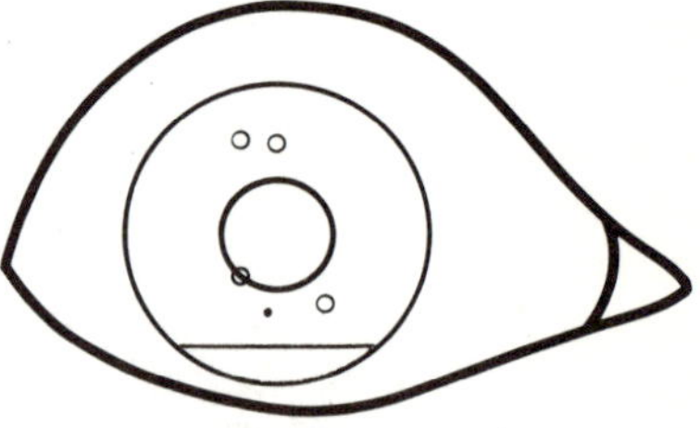

Fig. 5.3 Tuberculous nodules lying in the iris stroma with pus in the anterior chamber (a hypopyon) and a Koeppe nodule at the pupil margin

cences come into prominence, those found at the pupillary border being commonly known as Koeppe nodules, and those found on the face of the iris as floccules or efflorescences. These are more appropriate terms than nodules, for the latter infers a solid structure, whereas they consist of a more delicate, almost translucent formation, even when pigmented. Further changes are the characteristic increase in the protein content of the aqueous humour, so that the passage of light through it reveals particles, protein and cells (flare); there may even be pus in the anterior chamber (Fig. 5.3) and finally there are extensive posterior adhesions (synechiae) binding not only the pupillary margin, but any portion of the back of the iris, to the underlying anterior lens capsule. A fine vitreous haze is usually present, which, if the posterior uvea is involved, will increase until the details are obscured. In severe anterior uveitis cases, a secondary cataract and secondary glaucoma are possibilities. Those clinical signs are not specific for tuberculosis; they are found in all cases of granulomatous anterior uveitis, but they were first described historically in connection with this disease.

When a posterior uveitis exists, the recurrence of circumscribed 'daughter' lesions *contiguous to older, quiescent lesions,* leaves a characteristic picture, the distribution of which somewhat resembles that found in disseminated syphilitic posterior uveitis (syn. choroiditis), but the number of lesions is very much less. In addition, the individual lesions are usually larger. A solitary circumscribed tuberculous lesion covering the macula has been reported more than once, and when this happens, distinguishing this lesion from toxoplasmosis is extremely difficult. When, on the other hand, there are several lesions, the fact that in tuberculosis they are contiguous and in toxoplasmosis they may be adjacent, but not contiguous, is worth noting.

Recurrences of retinal and vitreous haemorrhages

This complication is possibly due to tuberculosis, but can also occur in sickle cell disease and as a result of a bacterial vasculitis. Recurrent haemorrhages occur from small vessels at the transitional zone between the posterior segment and the periphery; at first intraretinal, some may penetrate the vitreous. From early days this condition has been known as *Eales' disease.* Generally found in young adults,

recurrent bleeding leads in the end to seriously impaired sight. High blood pressure and diabetes must be excluded.

Optic neuritis

As a result of a tuberculous basal meningitis, as in syphilis, an optic neuritis is sometimes seen, usually without involvement of any of the extraocular nerves.

Treatment

Chemotherapy

It has not been established yet that ocular tuberculosis responds to standard courses of chemotherapy. Treatment of the eye has, therefore, of necessity, to be symptomatic.

Treatment of pulmonary tuberculosis in the tropics is handicapped by the high cost of rifampicin (a very important drug) and by the reluctance of patients to take the prescribed drugs for the full duration of the course. In the tropics 6 months inpatient treatment, or 18 months daily treatment, is frequently an impossible dream outside the facilities and control of patients in even the largest town.

Preventive therapy

Mass BCG vaccination programs are effective in helping to control tuberculosis in developing countries, but the benefits are not seen for several years. If mass BCG programs are to be used, they should be directed at children at or below the age of 5. In practice it is easier to arrange to give BCG by mouth at birth, when it is unnecessary to precede it with a pre-tuberculin test.

VARIOLA (SMALLPOX) AND VACCINIA

The diseases and their symptomatology

On 26th October, 1979, the World Health Organisation officially declared smallpox a disease having been brought under full control. Dr Jenner of Gloucestershire, when he introduced vaccination in 1796, would have been astounded to know that smallpox, once the scourge of Europe, as well as Afro-Asia, much to be feared in every tropical country up to the 1970s, would finally be brought under control by his discovery. Spread by a virus (*Poxvirus variolae*), a member of the group which includes vaccinia virus (*P. officinale*), cowpox virus (*P. bovis*) and others, variola results from droplet and touch transmission. *Vaccinia*, it is generally agreed, is smallpox which has been permanently modified by passage through the calf, probably as the result of a mutation. It is not a natural disease.

In 1978 WHO formed a Global Commission for the Certification of Smallpox Eradication, the terms of service being to review existing data, visit selected countries where smallpox had recently been endemic and make an objective assessment whether in fact it has been eradicated. The Commission concluded smallpox had been eradicated from India in 1977. The last Commission visit took place at the end of 1979 in the Horn of Africa where the last case had been recorded (in October 1977). No cases were found. In the belief that 2 years is sufficient to confirm the interruption of transmission, the findings of the last Commission would appear to be sufficient to confirm the final interruption of transmission. It is concluded the risk of its re-introduction is now negligible (Arita, 1979).

The smallpox virus enters the respiratory tract, invades and multiplies in the lymph nodes, thereby reaching the blood, from which it spreads throughout the reticuloendothelial system, in which it further multiplies; once again entering the blood, the virus reaches the skin and mucous membranes. The patient now has a high fever and is often comatose. Papules, vesicles, pustules and scabs form to produce the classical cutaneous appearance of smallpox. Death from toxaemia, helped along by secondary infection, used to kill many thousands. It also used to blind many thousands. *As the fear of a recrudescence of smallpox will be present for a long time, it is important in a sporadic case, when there is a rash, to differentiate it from chickenpox.* In smallpox the rash is scanty on the abdomen and chest, whereas in chickenpox it is as widespread there as on the face and back. In chickenpox the rash tends to avoid the limbs; in smallpox it is present on the limbs. The papules are circular, multilocular and umbilicated in smallpox, not so in chickenpox, where they are oval, never umbilicated and generally not multilocular. The papules in *both* diseases soften to become vesicles, then pustules, which ulcerate and scab over. All stages (papules, vesicles, pustules and scabs) are seen at any one time in chickenpox, but *in smallpox the lesions are of the same kind at each time of viewing.*

Ocular features

The pustules of smallpox can spread from the lids, which are grossly swollen, to the eyeball, producing membranous and sometimes haemorrhagic conjunctivitis, with a profuse discharge; corneal lesions ulcerate, hypopyon sometimes resulting, especially if a secondary infection supervenes. The corneal ulcer can perforate, leading to loss of the eye (endophthalmitis followed by phthisis). Alternatively, the ulcers may give rise to a deep and wide corneal abscess which, if it regresses and heals, leaves a dense leucoma; if the abscess perforates, a *leucoma adherens* (in which the iris has plugged the perforation) can result. The association of these changes, more usually bilateral than in measles, with the healed scabs of smallpox on the face and lids, is pathognomonic, a picture still seen in survivors.

Accidental vaccination of the lids with *P. officinale* is not uncommon. It results in the development of one or more serpiginous ulcers, which may be as wide as a finger. These very often enlarge until they encroach on the lid margins, and may be confused with fungal infections, but there are no serious systemic symptoms. The vaccinia ulcer has a raised white edge and the floor is covered with a thick, necrotic membrane, which when it falls off shows a raw, red surface (Plate 46). Healing is remarkably complete. The infection can spread to the conjunctiva and the cornea, but this is rare. Obviously lesions are far worse in those not previously vaccinated.

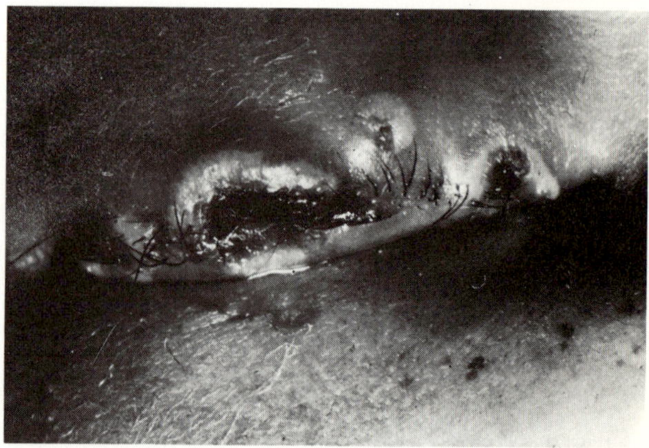

Plate 46 Vaccinia ulceration of upper lid

Corneal complications are said to arise in a third of those who have ulcers of the lids or face. In those subjects without a generalised variola, but a localised vaccinial cutaneous lid or face ulcer, involvement of the cornea usually presents as a punctate subepithelial keratitis, staining with Rose Bengal and somewhat resembling epidemic keratoconjunctivitis. The affected areas of the cornea may then break down and form a painful ulcer which stains and adopts a dendron-like shape, so that it may be mistaken for a dendritic ulcer; it is associated with an underlying stromal reaction. Later still, a deep stromal keratitis has been described, which consolidates into a disciform keratitis.

Treatment

Iodoxuridine 0.1 per cent eyedrops are effective in vaccinia keratitis, if applied 2-hourly for several days, and if not interrupted too quickly when a cure appears to have occurred; it is better to continue for a few days after healing. Idoxuridine 5 per cent lotion applied to the lid ulcers 4 times a day will promote fairly quick healing. Secondary infection should be checked with antibiotics, administered orally.

6

Rare tropical eye conditions

This chapter is one for quick reference. Some of the diseases might well have been placed in a previous chapter, for example, amoebiasis and rubella are very common. However, amoebiasis is not recognisable as such in an ophthalmic patient and the diagnosis is difficult to confirm; rubella causes embryopathic lesions in the fetus if the mother is infected during pregnancy, but the disease (which gives permanent immunity) is so common in childhood that this very seldom happens. The majority of the diseases listed here are rare.

In a few brief paragraphs at the start, the geographical distribution, cause and symptoms are given. The diagnoses, more than in any of the others, should benefit from laboratory back-up, even on the modest scale given in Chapter 7. The present chapter lists the diseases concerned under the headings of infectious diseases, the zoonoses, parasitic infestations and mycotic infections, and ends with some unusual ophthalmias. With it a description of the eye diseases most likely to be found in the tropics is completed.

INFECTIOUS DISEASES

Amoebiasis (amoebic dysentery)

Found in all tropical countries, the positive organism *Entamoeba histolytica* may live in the bowel without symptoms, or invade the bowel wall to produce dysentery, or spread to the liver and other organs; there seems no reason why it should not reach the eye. Nevertheless, there is still a great deal of doubt whether this does actually happen. Acute severe granulomatous anterior uveitis closely associated with amoebiasis has been reported many times, frequently responding to specific systemic treatment of the latter, but the association could be casual and the recovery spontaneous. A few cases of posterior (exudative) uveitis have also been reported and in a third small group in the USA a cystic lesion appeared at the fovea with adjacent haemorrhages, disappearing with antiamoebiasis treatment. The treatment has been revolutionised since the introduction of metronidazole (Flagyl).

Bacillary dysentery (shigellosis)

This infection, usually of the large intestine, is caused by the *Shigella* group: *Sh. dysenteriae* I and II *Sh. flexneri, Sh. boydii* and *Sh. sonnei,* the latter being the least severe. As the clinical symptoms vary from a mild diarrhoea to a severe toxic illness, so the range of ocular complications also varies, increasing with the severity of the dysentery; this in fact means that they are more usually associated with *Sh. dys. I (Shiga)*. The organisms are non-motile Gram-negative bacilli.

An exogenous keratoconjunctivitis, following touch-transmission, is always a possibility, as with any diarrhoea. A few cases of this have been reported; they respond to various antibiotics and the sulphonamides. More serious are reports of an associated anterior uveitis, but the nature of the uveitis is not clear, and with one exception they were reported during the First World War, and not since, so there must be some doubt about the authenticity of this aetiology, especially as it was frequently associated with arthritis and, in many instances, a urethritis. It sounds more like Reiter's syndrome, which one would expect to be common during a war. At any rate, uveitis as a complication of *Shigellosis* remains to be proven.

In small children attacks of bacillary dysentery may be the precipitating factor in xerophthalmia and keratomalacia. Reports of corneal ulceration in bacillary dysentery almost certainly refer to keratomalacia secondarily infected by direct faecal innoculation.

Treatment of gastroenteritis and in most cases bacillery dysentery should be conservative. Simple antidiarrhoeals such as Lomotil (Searle), should be used, and fluids and salt administered freely. Antibiotics are usually not indicated. Sulphadimidine may need to be administered where the response is slow.

Cholera

The cholera bacillus *(Vibrio cholerae)* is half as big as a tubercle bacillus. Its ravages have accounted for many pandemics from China to the Mediterranean and beyond. Apart from the obvious risk of exposure keratitis or corneal abrasions when the lids of a collapsed patient remain partially open, the tears participating in a general dehydration being minimal, there are four types of 'red eye' reported from pandemic areas: congested eyes, an acute conjunctivitis, linear corneal ulcers with conjunctivitis, and corneal oedema. The last may be due to an upset of osmolarity of the serum, so that the cornea holds fluid and electrolytes more than normally. It is believed an upset of osmolarity is the basis for the onset of total (black) cataract, which can develop in the extreme stages of cholera, as indeed it can in the last stages of any dehydrating infectious disease. Tetracycline and Chloramphenicol are equally effective drugs, but there are ominous rumblings that resistant strains of *vibrio cholerae* are developing.

Lymphogranuloma venereum (Nicolas-Favré disease)

The positive agent of this universal disease is a typical member of the group of micro-organisms called *Chlamydia* (which includes the TRIC agent described in Chap. III). These viruses cannot be differentiated morphologically, only by their clinical manifestations. Although distribution is worldwide, the ocular complications are more common in negroes and Latin Americans. The primary lesion (a small sore) is usually genital, associated with a regional lymphadenitis. The primary lymphogranuloma arises rarely on the lids.

A severe follicular conjunctivitis sometimes arises following finger transference, and may end up affecting the whole eye. General dissemination (wherein the virus penetrates the monocytes or polymorph leucocytes within the blood) can lead to diffuse marginal corneal ulcers with associated dilated vessels, which may enter the cornea; corneal infiltration localised in upper or lower sectors also occurs. These appearances have been described as 'epaulets'; the keratitis extends inwards with new (superficial) vessels in attendance, which colour the opacity. Diagnosis has been confirmed by virus isolation, so there is no question as to the authenticity of this ocular lesion.

An anterior uveitis in the tertiary stage has been described by a few writers, but the association may be incidental, as in each case it was a granulomatous uveitis, almost unknown in viral infections. Moreover, there were other changes suggestive of Behcet's or Reiter's syndromes.

In some 5 per cent of tertiary stage cases, retinal vascular dilations and tortuosity, with or without an exudative retinitis and haemorrhages, have been reported and supported by histopathologies which demonstrated typical intraocular cytomegalic inclusion cells.

Treatment is symptomatic to the eye. Oral sulphonamides give good results in early cases. Tetracyclines, and oxytetracycline in particular, should be used if sulphonamides fail.

Relapsing fever (louse-borne)

Relapsing fever is another spirochaete infection caused by an organism called *Borrellia* (sometimes called *Treponema*) *recurrentis,* transmitted by lice. In the louse-borne variety of relapsing fever man is the only host, and so epidemics may occur through the repetitive bites of the vector. The tick vector feeds on animals and man, preferably the latter, and is discussed under the heading of 'Zoonoses'. *B. recurrentis* is found in the body fluids and blood vessels. Being neurotropic, it may affect the meninges and central nervous system. *B. duttoni* normally is tick-borne, but there is some evidence that it can infect lice as well.

The ocular lesions are variable and are associated with the presence of *B. recurrentis* in the peripheral blood. They include a mild interstitial keratitis, occurring late, acute anterior granulomatous uveitis with marked exudates in the posterior chamber, a chronic anterior uveitis, and rarely a posterior uveitis. Optic neuritis has also been reported. It is likely that direct invasion of each structure occurs. In about one quarter of cases the condition is bilateral. These lesions are seldom seen in the early recurring fevers. It may be associated with a palsy of one or other of the extraocular muscles in late, severe cases.

The tetracyclines are most effective.

Rubella (German measles)

German measles is a mild virus illness, spread by droplet infection. No specific treatment is required. The distribution is worldwide, but in the tropics so common is it in childhood that mothers are only rarely infected during pregnancy. The worst effect is on the defenceless fetus of a mother suffering from the disease. The virus strikes the fetus within the first 3 months of pregnancy. As it may persist for several months after infection, a mother, infected recently before pregnancy, puts the fetus at risk, although not as greatly as when actually suffering from rubella during the first 3 months of pregnancy. (For this reason the vaccine, being an attenuated living rubella, should not be given to pregnant women, nor for 3 months *before* pregnancy if possible.)

It has been established that where the mother is infected during the first 3 months of pregnancy there is a 10 to 20 per cent chance the child will be stillborn or born with a variety of teratogenic anomalies; the eye, ear, heart and brain are particularly affected. There is nothing that can be done if this situation presents itself before the child is born.

The ocular changes, affecting one or both eyes, include an embryopathic cataract (nuclear, atypical or total), frequently with a small pupil in a small eye (microphthalmos). Less commonly buphthalmos has also been reported, as has strabismus, iris deformities, corneal opacities and congenital glaucoma. *It should be remembered that high intraocular pressure is an epiphenomenon in the newborn for several weeks.* Another defect which can confuse, where everything else seems in perfect order and where there is no positive history of rubella in the mother, is a pigmentary degeneration of the retina, which can simulate a luetic 'pepper and salt' fundus, a primary retinitis pigmentosa, secondary pigmentary degeneration after an arterial occlusion (usually sectorial), and any early central or paracentral macular change.

The classic finding in rubella is a centrally placed dispersal of fine pigment granules around the macular area, with loss of central vision and nystagmus. This is discussed in Chapter 4 at greater length.

Surgery for cataract, done within a year when the virus may still be present, does badly; an anterior uveitis invariably complicates the operation. Treatment otherwise is symptomatic.

Typhoid fever

The *Salmonellae* which cause the enteric group of fevers—typhoid and paratyphoids A, B and C—are Gram-negative bacilli, with numerous flagellae. They can be identified only by various laboratory techniques which demonstrate their individual characteristics. The distribution is global, but typhoid fever is particularly common in the tropics, and it is *S. typhi* (typhoid) which is associated with eye lesions, not paratyphoid. The spread of infection is from man to man via water, food or flies. Symptom-free carriers are common.

Rose spots on the conjunctiva have been reported many times. Uveal complications through the invasion of *S. typhi* are rare. In epidemics, as with many acute fevers, bilateral cataracts have been reported in severe cases. As they appear in those who are most toxic, a minority only survives. A secondary retinitis pigmentosa has been observed, but as only one such case has been reported since 1960, this is perhaps doubtful. Pupillary and extraocular muscle palsies occur without doubt when there is perivascular invasion of the central nervous system in the seriously ill. These defects are frequently permanent.

Chloramphenicol, despite some toxic side effects, is the drug of choice.

Typhus fever (louse-borne)

This disease (with trench fever) is the only fever caused by the genus *Rickettsia* which is not a zoonosis. It has a global distribution. Typhus carried by the body louse is the classical typhus of urban epidemics and is much less likely to be seen than rural tick-borne or mite-borne, or the comparatively mild flea-borne (murine) typhus in the tropics. The latter insects having intermediate animal hosts are all described in the next section (the zoonoses).

The organism responsible for louse-borne typhus

is *Rickettsia prowazeki*. The infection reaches man mainly by louse faeces, through the skin or rarely the external ocular membranes.

Small, oval, pink-purple spots on the conjunctiva (not dissimilar to the rose spots of typhoid) in association with a body rash and disappearing with it, have been reported. Keratoconjunctivitis may also occur and be more prolonged. Subconjunctival haemorrhages of varying sizes are common. During an epidemic the *cataracta cachectica,* described already in several acute toxic infections (cholera, typhoid, etc), may arise. An anterior uveitis, more rarely a posterior, with or without retinal haemorrhages and a central serous retinopathy, has been described, as has retinal venous thrombosis, usually of a branch vessel. Despite meningeal irritation, involvement of the ocular cranial nerves has never been described, although in the zoonotic typhuses they have. Late relapses of louse-borne typhus (Brill-Zinsser disease) have not been associated with any of the above changes other than the conjunctival, and then only occasionally.

Chloramphenicol and the tetracyclines are highly specific.

THE ZOONOSES

Brucellosis (undulant fever)

Three species of the genus *Brucella* are involved: *Br. melitensis, Br. abortus* and *Br. suis.* They are Gramnegative coccoid bacilli and are non-motile. *Brucella* as a general rule is transmitted to man from animals by ingestion, by direct or indirect contact via the lungs or through the external ocular membranes. It is widely distributed both in the temperate and tropical areas of the world.

In the early stages pain on movement of the eyes (due to a tenonitis, not an optic neuritis) is common. Invasion of the orbit can lead to single oculomotor palsies. A brucellar basal meningoencephalitis can cause bilateral sixth nerve paralysis, the latter being particularly vulnerable by reason of its long course.

Clinical and experimental evidence indicates that coin-shaped subepithelial opacities in the cornea (nummular keratitis) occur in brucellosis. These opacities remain a long time before becoming absorbed.

The *Brucella* organisms have never been conclu-

sively demonstrated in the uvea of an eye with uveitis. The experimental and clinical evidence, on the other hand, makes it highly probable. In those suffering from the chronic phase, recurrent granulomatous anterior uveitis arises. Definite nodules are not seen on the surface of the iris, but there is a suggestion that they exist deep in the stroma, indicated by undulations on the surface. The lardaceous KP are small. The posterior uveitis of brucellosis is equally nonspecific, consisting of several moderately-sized areas of exudation with very little surrounding reaction. Those described are either polyhedral or trapezoid in shape. The inflammation is self-limiting, leaving behind pigmented scars.

The best treatment in the acute phase is obtained by an intensive course of tetracycline and sulphadiazine. In the chronic stage the condition reacts best to a specific vaccine (Woods, 1961).

Tularaemia is usually discussed with brucellosis, as the causative organism is a *Brucella, Br. (pasturella) tularensis,* a short Gramnegative rod. It is transmitted from rodents, in which it is a natural infection, to man by the bite of a variety of infected insects, by touching infected animals or by taking infected water. However, tularaemia has not been found in the tropics. It occurs as a human infection in North America, Europe (including the USSR) and Japan. The lids are commonly swollen and reddened. Parinaud's oculoglandular syndrome is one of the main clinical types of tularaemia.

Leishmaniasis

Caused by flagellate protozoa of the genus *Leishmania* (such as *L. donovani, tropica, etc.*) initially, perhaps solely, animal parasites, this disease now spreads either by man–fly–man or animal–fly–man transmission, by several *Phlebotomine* sandflies. It is a chronic, infective disease, usually although not entirely a zoonosis, causing cutaneous lesions or, more severely, systemic (visceral), with hepatosplenomegaly and irregular fever and leucopenia, especially in young males and children. The visceral form (kala-azar) varies greatly in its complexity and severity in different parts of the world.

Visceral leishmaniasis with a rodent reservoir

The sandfly, *Phlebotomus argentipes,* is the principal vector and feeds solely on man. Epidemics have occurred at irregular intervals. The organism is *L. donovani*. It is found in India, Bangladesh and Assam.

Visceral leishmaniasis with a rodent reservoir

Strains of *Leishmania* are found south of the Sahara in Africa, in Eritrea and Ethiopia and in South Sudan. It is transmitted by *P. orientalis* in the Sudan and *P. martini* in West Africa. When epidemics occur, transmission is by man–fly–man, and it is no longer a zoonosis; but this is rare.

Visceral leishmaniasis with a canine reservoir

L. donovani is found in the Mediterranean littoral as well as in Western, Eastern and Central Asia, part of China and in Central and Southern America. It occurs in both man and dogs, including jackals, especially the latter. The various phlebotomine vectors involved are both anthropo- and zo-ophilic. Children are particularly liable to infection. This is strictly a zoonosis, although man–fly–man transmission may occur usually during epidemics.

In the Old World (e.g. India) a primary leishmanioma (oriental sore) forms at the site of a bite infected by *L. tropica*. Usually they are quite small. In the New World (e.g. Brazil) expanding cutaneous lesions (espundia) are widespread; they are caused by one of the *L. braziliensis* strains. An immune system develops in the course of the primary lesion, during which some of the organisms get into the blood and circulate or come to rest in the reticuloendothelial system. Here, within the cells, they multiply until the cells either seal or rupture, and the flagellate parasites spread further in the blood through the viscera (kala-azar), a stage which can be fatal if untreated.

When leishmaniasis infects the viscera, as stated above, it is a serious disease; however, it is essentially a mucocutaneous infection and the lesion of the skin (known as 'oriental sore' in Afro-Asia, and 'espundia' in Central and South America) is a chronic infection, sometimes remaining dry (as in oriental sore), and therefore, chronic; at other times it suppurates (as in espundia), and in consequence becomes more extensive and destructive. Early on, it resembles lepromatous leprosy (Plate 47).

In addition to mutilations of the lids, and the face, it is not infrequent to find the conjunctiva of the lids

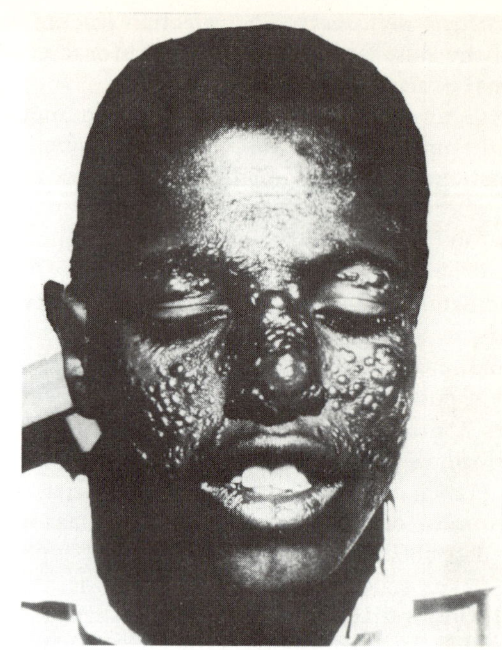

Plate 47 Leishmaniasis of face and upper lids

secondarily involved, presenting as a granular (papilliform) conjunctivitis. There follows a superficial, then stromal, coin-shaped collection of opacities in the cornea, with new vessels growing inwards towards them. There is now pain, photophobia and lacrimation. Although multiple lesions of the skin are the rule, one attack generally confers immunity. In visceral leishmaniasis (kala-azar), despite the fact that the parasites have spread widely in the blood into the spleen, liver and large intestine, there is great doubt if they ever infect the inner eye. As there is an anaemia and leucopenia and fever, retinal haemorrhages may be seen; reports are few and far between.

The pentavalent antimony preparations are the drugs of choice for treatment. Retinal exudates (kala-azar retinopathy) have been reported in cases of dermal leishmanoid responding to this treatment.

Leptospirosis (swamp fever)

The causative organism is a motile, spiral organism of the genus *Leptospira*. It is found worldwide. The relationships of the principal hosts of *Leptospira* involve rats, cattle, horses, pigs, dogs and so on, and is most confusing; it is a highly complex zoonosis. Man may become infected by bites or by touching the skin, nose, mouth or external eyes of the hosts. The disease usually ends in man. The *Leptospira interrogans* complex (with several strains) is pathogenic for man and animals. When the symptoms, usually mild or moderate, become severe and fatal, although this is not a separate condition, it was (initially) described as *Weil's disease*, and this term has stuck, although it is not synonymous with leptospirosis.

The organisms invade the eye and may be present in the aqueous after they have gone from the blood, which occurs in about a week. An anterior uveitis arises when immunity has faded, although this takes time. The usual time of onset is about 6 months after the disease has passed, and the complication is quite common. It may present as a chronic granulomatous uveitis, or as an acute nongranulomatous associated with a high agglutinin titre, an allergic reaction.

Clouding of the vitreous indicates involvement of the posterior uvea, the same delay in its onset occurring as with the anterior uvea. Exudates and haemorrhages in the retina and optic nerve are also described at this stage along with the formation of veils of a fibrinous exudate, extending especially from the optic nerve into the vitreous. Despite the menacing appearance of the posterior uveitis, it more often than not runs a mild course and recovers well, although the veils can persist for several years.

In the severe, acute variety (Weil's disease), as additional features, an intense conjunctival congestion with subconjunctival haemorrhages is seen, and jaundice may discolour the sclera.

High doses of antibiotics are indicated, especially penicillin.

Relapsing fever (tick-borne)

Discussed already in the previous section as an infectious fever, spread from man to man by lice, the tick-borne variety differs by reason of the fact that it feeds on certain animals (in which the disease is a natural infection), such as rodents, monkeys, squirrels and probably bats, and the tick can pass the infection on to man if by chance it bites him; alternatively, if the tick alights on man, as its secretions are infected the organisms can penetrate intact mucous membranes and skin without the tick biting. With such a varied natural history sporadic cases are to be expected, not epidemics.

The disease is transmitted by soft ticks of the genus *Ornithodorus,* which live in warm climates such as southern Europe, Afro-Asia, Central and South America and the Near East. *Borrellia recurrentis* does not infect ticks, only lice. Other species of *Borellia* infect ticks in the tropics, such as *B. duttoni* in Africa and *B. venezuelensis* in Central and South America.

An anterior uveitis is said to occur, but is doubtful in the case of tick-borne infections. When a meningitis results with infections of *B. duttoni,* ophthalmoplegias, facial paralysis, papillitis and optic atrophy have all been reported.

The tetracyclines are effective curatives.

Toxocariasis

Toxocara canis and *cati* are common nematodes in puppies and cats. Infection in man is acquired by accidental ingestion of eggs from animal faeces. The disease is worldwide. It is far more common in young children than in adults. The eggs hatch out in the child's upper intestine and the larvae migrate into the blood, lymphatics and tissue spaces; the larvae (there are four stages) never mature into adult worms in man and can probably remain alive only for a matter of months. If the final resting place is in the eye it can produce blindness. The size of the organism probably seldom exceeds 50 μm.

Toxocara granulomas containing dead larvae and many eosinophilic leucocytes have been found in the orbit.

If the anterior uvea is affected-without posterior uveal involvement-by a *toxocara larva,* there is usually only a mild reaction; subacute inflammation is the rule. However, an exudative posterior uveitis (Plate 48), with or without an associated granulomatous anterior inflammation, has been described in association with a disintegrating larva and can be serious.

The early retinal changes when the posterior segment of the eye is invaded by a larva have been recently described by Dean Hart & Raistrick (1977). The retinas exhibit linear reflexes, which change position if viewed over a period of days (larva migrans). A raised pigmented lesion may suddenly become apparent, surrounded by oedema. Deeper, discrete retinal haemorrhages are frequently associated. The elevated lesion in time settles and changes into a pale, circular umbilicated oedematous mass, into which a dilated retinal vessel, or vessels,

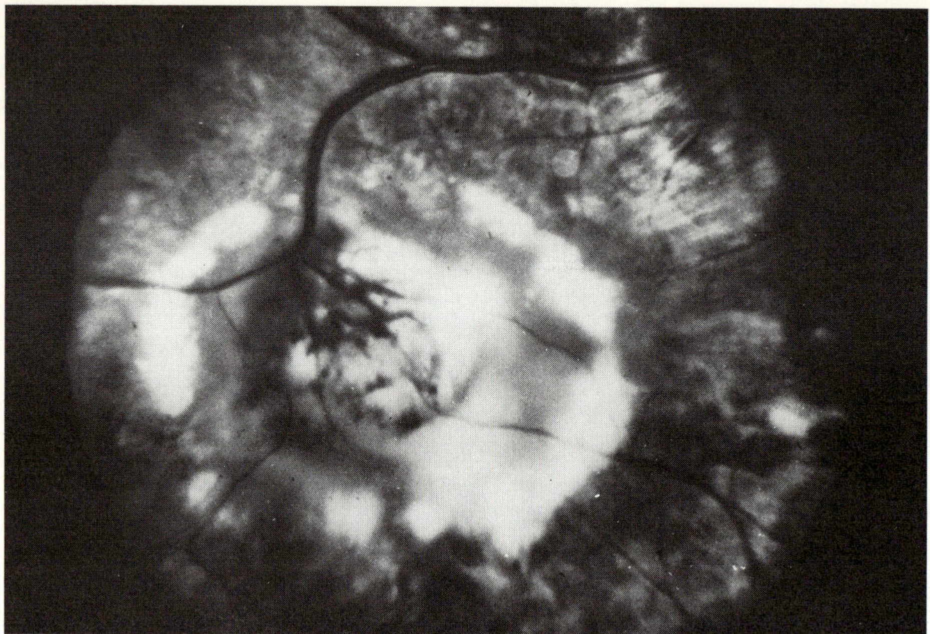

Plate 48 Toxocariasis of posterior uvea involving the macula

frequently dips. When the retinal oedema disappears, persistent pigmentary disturbance and heaped-up gliosis beome more obvious. The differential diagnosis should include Coats' disease, endophthalmitis and retinoblastoma.

The treatment of this disease is with diethylcarbamazine, but whether the disease is fully arrested or not by this drug is a little uncertain.

Toxoplasmosis

The presence of *Toxoplasma gondii* in man in tropical countries, as well as in the West, has been increasingly reported in congenital form. In the acquired form this is not the case; it is still extremely rare. *T. gondii* has a (coccidial) life cycle in the intestines of cats, dogs, monkeys etc. The eggs are excreted in their faeces and transmitted to man, probably by ingestion or droplet spread. The disease may affect one or both eyes. The organism is a protozoa (Sporozoa) and stains with Giemsa. The trophozoites (4 to 6 μm in length) and the cysts (100 μm) are the only phases that have been found in man.

In eye congenital form, the organisms acquired by the fetus from maternal blood reach the choroid via the blood vessels. Mostly they then enter the retina, for which they have a liking, and in that structure they are contained within a cyst. They produce a localised chorioretinitis, which heals spontaneously, but leaves a scar with destruction of the neuroretinal elements. Mothers are carriers without a symptomatology. Children having acquired the infection late in the mother's pregnancy seem to be those most affected. In some 80 per cent of cases the focal chorioretinal scar is uniocular. It may be peripheral, but unfortunately in many affects the macula. This lesion should always be sought if an infant is seen to have a squint in a blind eye. Later damage, due to the bursting of cysts with the spread of the infection and formation of secondary (daughter) lesions, usually occurs, if at all, in the first and second decades. If they are seen in adults, then the diagnosis is more questionable. All the foci end up (close together but separate, unlike tubercular chorioretinitis) as rounded, well circumscribed, pigmented scars of varying sizes, depths and degrees of pigmentation. Relapses cause acute oedematous reactions in the retina with vitreous haze (a choroiditis), which when they settle, are seen to have adopted a characteristic round pigmented scar configuration.

In the acquired form of toxoplasmosis there may be a typhus-like fever, or a meningoencephalitis,

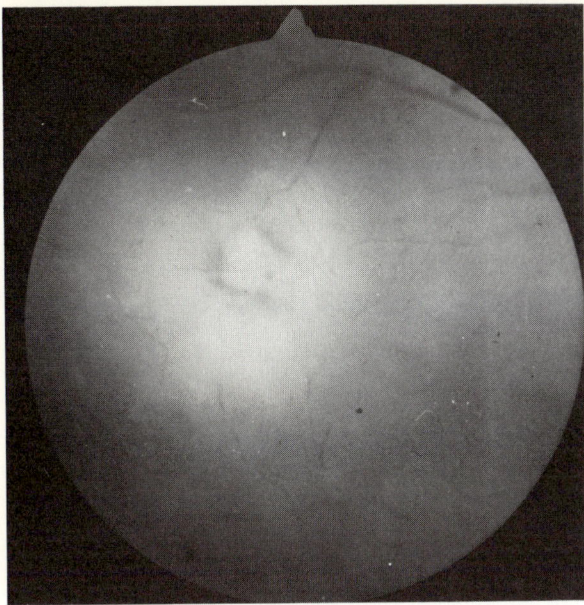

Plate 49 Adult toxoplasmosis initial chorioretinal focus

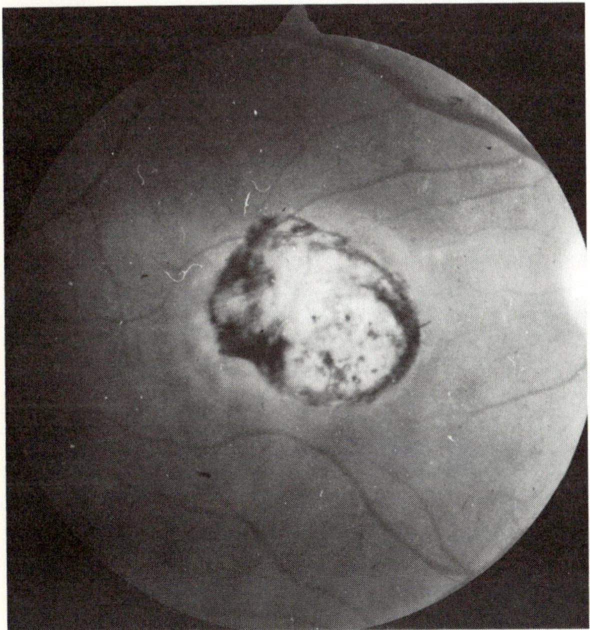

Plate 50 Same lesion as previous plate, healed

frequently mild. More commonly there is a lymphadenopathy, which may either be associated with a fever, or be asymptomatic. The uvea may be involved at this stage. The lesions attributed to acquired toxoplasmosis are a focal chorioretinitis

(Plates 49 and 50), somewhat like tuberculosis, an acute involvement of the entire uvea and a haemorrhagic perivasculitis of the retinal vessels, especially the veins. The anterior uveitis is classically a granulomatous one with large mutton fat KP and nodules in the stroma. Secondary (daughter) lesions in the posterior segment form around the original, as in the congenital form.

Treatment is with pyrimethamine given in tablet form plus sulphonamides in full dosage for 28 days along with Folinic acid supplement.

Typhus fever (tick-, mite- and flea-borne)

These are all *Rickettsia* fevers. Flea-borne (murine) typhus, except in the aged, is usually a mild disease conveyed to man by fleas which normally live on rodents.

In tick typhus a household dog is the preferred host. The disease is present in South, West and East Africa and in India as well as in the Mediterranean area. The mortality rate is negligible. The eye is not known to have been affected.

Mite-borne *scrub typhus* is acquired when man disturbs the scrub country in endemic areas; it is the variety most likely to be seen in man in the tropics and is caused by *Rickettsia orientalis,* a parasite of rodents. It is transmitted by a larval mite which attaches itself at random to birds, reptiles, rodents or man for a few days at a time. Thus, the infection is transmitted in the end from these creatures to man.

The tick-borne variety found in North and South America, more commonly called *'spotted fever'* had a generally high death rate until vaccines became available. It is caused by a virulent strain of *Rickettsia* (*R. rickettsi rickettsi*).

The ocular changes found in *scrub typhus* and *spotted fever* include a catarrhal conjunctivitis as well as congestion and photophobia in acute cases. In about 5 per cent there are subconjunctival haemorrhages which can be massive. The primary eschar (initial ulcer) has been seen on the lid. A very few cases of severe bilateral anterior granulomatous uveitis have been reported; by far the most frequent intraocular complications seen have been papilloedema, engorged retinal veins with haemorrhages, papillitis, and most common of all, optic neuritis, which can be followed by optic atrophy with field defects. Invasion of the central nervous system in severe cases produces thrombotic lesions, leading to oculomotor palsies in the febrile period. If such a patient survives, the palsy will probably persist.

Chloramphenicol and the tetracyclines are highly specific.

PARASITIC INFESTATIONS

Ancylostomiasis (ankylostomiasis, hookworm)

Ancylostoma duodenale and *Necator americanus* are nematodes (or round worms) which may be present in vast numbers in the small intestine of man. All tropical and subtropical countries are infested with one or other of them. As the name suggests, *N. americanus* is found in the Americas (save for Paraguay, Peru and Chile), but it is also the predominant hookworm in Central and South Africa, South Asia and the Caribbean. *A. duodenale* accounts for the rest of the tropical world, including Paraguay, Peru and Chile, apparently introduced there by Japanese fishermen.

Eggs discharged in the faeces of man develop into infective larvae in the soil in and around villages. They can bore through the skin of a new host, or accidentally be ingested. Those that bore through man's skin enter the blood and lymphatics, and after passively reaching the lungs, actively migrate via the capillaries, and by way of the bronchial tree reach the oesophagus, and being swallowed so reach their goal, the intestines. Chronic infections lead to blood loss with anaemia and vague abdominal symptoms. It is a most debilitating disease.

Ocular complications are rare. Perhaps as a result of the iron deficiency anaemia the parasites produce, *night blindness* is not infrequently associated with hookworm. Irritation due to endotoxins followed by hypersensitivity causes oedema of the lids, which may be the first indication of infection. The eye has not been seen clinically invaded by larvae or adult worms, but Wilder (1951) found the larvae in the chorioretina of 24 out of 46 eyes enucleated from young children with a mistaken clinical diagnosis of retinoblastoma. Eosinophilic granulomas in the vitreous with central necrosis were found in some of the eyes which she examined to contain hookworm larvae, either entire or disintegrating; in others the larvae were those of *Toxocara canis*. Migration tracks in the choroid and retina have subsequently been demonstrated, both histopathologically and by fluor-

escein angiography. The differential diagnosis of a local eosinophilic granuloma includes not only toxocara and retinoblastoma, but cysticercosis, Coats' disease and bacterial endophthalmitis.

The clinical association between hookworm and an exudative haemorrhagic lesion of the retina had been noted for some time before the findings of Wilder, but was considered to be due to an endotoxaemia, not the presence of hookworm larvae *per se*. Debilitation in children due to ancylostomiasis may trigger off xerophthalmia.

Strongyloides stercoralis is another extremely common nematode with a slightly different life history from the two described above. Mojon (1977) by serodiagnosis using the indirect fluorescent antibody test (and excluding the lower dilutions where cross reactions may exist) found that just under 80 per cent revealed infection, whereas in stool examinations of the same people the larvae were found in only 8 per cent. Despite its frequency and wide distribution—especially where there is moisture in addition to heat—and despite the fact that the life history within man parallels *Ancylostoma* and *Necator* (none having any need of an intermediate host) and despite the fact that at all stages the larva is about the size of the common hookworm, it has never been seen to affect or invade the eye.

Treatment of ancylostomiasis is by tetrachlorethylene or bephenium hydroxynaphthoate. Thiabendazole is very effective against strongyloidiasis, less so against ancylostomiasis.

Ascariasis (the common roundworm)

Ascaris lumbricoides is said possibly to infect one in every four of the world's population (Wilcocks & Manson-Bahr, 1972). It is the largest nematode to infest the small intestine of man. Whereas the others range from 2 to 12 mm, Ascaris females may reach 45 *cm*. The eggs pass out in man's faeces, infecting the soil, crops and vegetables. Ascariasis has a worldwide distribution, although the prevalence rate varies; in parts of Africa 90 to 100 per cent of the population are infected.

The clinical symptoms are partially related to the number of larvae present and partly to the organs invaded. The eggs swallowed by man hatch out in his intestines. The larvae then wander through the wall of the intestinal tract into lymphatics or veins. They pass in this way to the liver and right side of the heart, and from there may reach the eye. Hypersensitivity to *ascaris* is well recognised, so the pathogenesis of the ocular lesions depends on two factors common to most parasitic infestations, namely direct invasion by the adult or the larva and hypersensitivity (probably to an ascaridotoxin from a live larva), and the death of a larva *in situ,* as in ancylostomiasis.

The lids can swell in recurring cycles. Small adults have been recovered, rarely, from under the conjunctiva, but they do not affect the cornea. Ocular changes are largely posterior. It has been claimed, but not proven, that a severe granulomatous anterior uveitis can occur as a result of larval invasion of and death in the iris. Wandering *ascaris* larvae have, however, been found in the retina by more than one observer. Their presence may be associated with oedema and small haemorrhages. If the larva dies within the eye a localised reaction occurs and pigment cells from the retinal pigment epithelium migrate to surround the disintegrating body. The larva migrans of *Ascaris lumbricoides* at its longest is about 2.5 mm, and should not be confused with the larva of *O. volvulus,* hookworm or Toxocara, which are all under 350 μm long; but it can be confused with a small growing adult *O. volvulus.* Other larvae which enter the posterior segment of the eye, such as cysticercus and fly maggots, are very much bigger (5 to 20 mm).

Hookworm larvae cannot be treated. Piperazine and tetrachlorethylene kill the adults, as does bephenium hydroxynaphthoate.

Cysticercosis (larval taeniasis)

The larva of the (cestode) pork tapeworm, *Taenia solium,* is called *Cysticercus cellulosae.* It can damage the eye badly. Cysticercosis (as the presence of such larvae is designated) is found in all tropical countries and the USA. There is a vast literature concerning it. The adult worms are from 2 to 3 metres long. The eggs are swallowed by man in infected meat or accidentally by touch-transmission and hatch in the stomach or duodenum, from whence the motile larvae reach various resting places via the mesenteric vessels. They may also, by entering the respiratory tree, reach the laryngopharyngeal area and be re-swallowed to grow into new adults in the intestines of the host. In about 2 months larvae which have not reached the intestinal tract form cysticerci. A cysticercus may be described as a small larva with an invaginated scolex and neck, a miniature adult. They produce a fibrocellular reaction wherever they come to rest, and will become calcified (so are radio-opaque) after death. The size varies with their age (5 to 20 mm)

Cysticerci have been found in the upper lids and orbit as small, soft, pea-shaped masses under the conjunctiva (mostly near the inner canthus), as well as the anterior uvea. An anterior uveitis with secondary glaucoma has been reported several times. The larva can remain alive and active for many months in the anterior chamber, the vitreous humor, below the subhyaloid membrane of the retina, i.e. *in* the retina, or under the neuroretina and in the subretinal space. A vitreo- or anterior-chamber cysticercus is seen as a rounded mass with iridescent edges, within which is a chalky white central spot, the scolex.

When present in the anterior chamber or vitreous cavity there is remarkably little reaction: a low grade inflammation, slight preretinal fibrosis or a few posterior lens changes (Plate 51). Below the neuroretina it can be seen as a slowly undulating mass, perhaps associated with exudates or haemorrhages. As it grows and migrates from there, the cysticercus may tear the retina. However, only if it dies does it seem to cause a severe reaction, which is localised. Rarely, it has apparently become encapsulated in life by glial and fibrous tissue within the retina, and there is no gross reaction around this lesion. The debris of the degenerate parasite has been identified in pathological sections.

Kende (1970) working in Mexico records 70 cases out of some 64 000 surgical patients seen over a 6-year period, roughly one case of cysticercosis a month. The distribution was as follows:

Lids	1
Anterior chamber	3
Subconjunctiva	7
Vitreous	28
Subretina	31

Surgical removal from the anterior chamber directly, or from the subretina via the posterior route, requires high technical ability. There is no effective alternative, apart from the symptomatic.

Dracontiasis (Guinea worm)

Dracunculus medinensis, a somatic roundworm or

nematode, has a special prevalence in limited districts within certain parts of Africa and India, the Valley of the Nile and Americas. It is widespread in Afro-Asia among carnivores. The female Guinea worm lies in the subcutaneous tissue of the limbs or trunk. It may be 60 cm in length. In 85 per cent of subjects this roundworm presents in the lower extremities. When man washes himself in infected water, the female worm within his extremities pierces the skin and discharges the embryos. If the intermediate host, *Cyclops,* is present in the water, they take up the embryos, and later man becomes infected by swallowing this micro-crustacean.

Immature Guinea worms have been dissected out from the upper lids several times, perhaps several at one time. Usually, however, they are single. They have also been found under the conjunctiva. It is strange that they should sometimes go against the rule and move towards the upper limbs and head. They have also been found in the orbit. There is no insect host, and larval forms are not found in the blood or subcutaneous tissue.

The gravid Guinea worm should not at the first sign of it be pulled out from the skin. It breaks easily. Daily douching over 10 days or so will cause the uterus to be emptied and the worm to protrude a little more on each occasion, after which it can be gently expressed or withdrawn if the worm has not done so spontaneously.

Diethylcarbamazine is believed to kill the worm as the general erythema and congestion of the eyes, which is asociated with its presence, is soon reduced following such treatment.

Echinococcosis (hydatid disease)

The accidental invasion of man's body by a cestode larva was illustrated by the larva of *Taenia solium* (cysticercosis). *Echinococcus* is another example. The genus is worldwide. The adult *E. granulosus* or *Taenia echinococcus* is quite small, consisting of only four segments, its total length being no more than 9 mm. An encysted larva is known as a hydatid cyst and can grow to 10 cm in diameter. It leads a separate existence like the cysticercus. The dog is the optimum definitive host, becoming infected by eating the infected meat of an intermediate host such as the ox. It is the dog's excreta which is the source of the eggs swallowed by man, in whom the hydatid cyst will later develop. After 3 months in man the cysts are 5 cm in diameter, and after another 5 or 6 weeks they can become 10 cm in diameter, or more.

The presence of a hydatid cyst has been reported only once or twice within the eye, but they are not uncommon in the orbit. The subjects are usually under 30. It increases in size over a period of months, and may in the end project out of the orbit. By this time the cyst may be as large as the eyeball itself, and the latter becomes displaced. Within the eye, the hydatid is subretinal and simulates a choroidal tumour.

The cysts have to be removed surgically. Treatment otherwise is symptomatic.

Gnathostomiasis

The adult stages of *Gnathostoma spinigerum,* another round worm, are normally found in nodules in the stomachs of wild and domestic animals, especially felines; in man they exist only as larvae, which survive, but not being adapted to the human body, wander aimlessly as immature worms in the subcutaneous tissues. Eggs evacuated by the host animal into water, hatch out and are reingested (as in the case of Guinea worm) by a microcrustacean, *Cyclops.* They emerge into water from the crustacean as second stage larvae, to be eaten by fish, frogs or snakes, in which they are converted into third stage larvae; any one of the intermediate hosts may be eaten by a dog or cat, or by man, especially if the latter eats poorly processed or undercooked fish. Man cannot be infected by eating the crustacean or by drinking infected water, for the first and second stage larvae do not survive in the stomach juices. This disease is common in the Far East, in Thailand, Vietnam, Malaysia and East Africa.

As does the adult of *Loa loa,* so the larva of *G. spinigerum* migrates under the skin, leaving a track of subsiding oedema in its wake. There are episodes of swelling, lasting up to a week, and the larva appears to be able to live for 10 years. Ocular complications have been reported; a third stage larva (3 mm) has been removed from the anterior chamber and identified. Its presence was associated with a granulomatous uveitis. It has not, strangely enough, been seen under the conjunctiva. A few cases of invasion of the eye by the posterior route are on record, but more proof is needed to be quite certain of this.

There is no treatment apart from removal of the worms.

Ophthalmomyiasis

Ophthalmomyiasis is a term used to describe infestation of the human eye by maggots (larvae) which come from various flies in the order of *Diptera*. Known hosts include cattle, sheep, horses, deer and man himself. They are as common in the West as they are in tropical countries. In addition to flies, vectors such as ticks and mosquitoes can convey the eggs of some of them to man; man-to-man touch transmission is also a factor. The most common ocular lesions are associated with those flies which, like the bots, prefer to deposit their larvae on the moist lid margins. The size of the maggots varies from 10 to 30 mm.

Larval infestation of the external ocular membranes or the orbit has been not infrequently reported and may result from the parasites being dropped into the eye when the fly is in flight. Apart from the usual signs of an irritable eye, the maggots themselves can be found in the upper or lower fornices and are quite difficult to remove. Screw-worm and other maggots may burrow beneath the conjunctiva, forming small undulating nodules, which on death give rise to granulomas. They may also penetrate the sclera, probably taking advantage of the easier access afforded by the perforating ciliary vessels; they then can give rise to an anterior uveitis, or worse, with much pain. Within the retina, if they reach there, they have been known to cause detachment, and, if subretinal, often become encysted. Free-floating in the vitreous, maggots cause least pain and distress; they may ultimately die *in situ*, but vision usually is lost, or diminished. The species most frequently involved are as follows:

1. *Cuterebridae:*
    a. *Dermatobia hominis* (tropical warble fly), found in tropical South and Central America

2. *Calliphoridae:*
    a. *Cordylobia anthropophaga* (the tumbu fly), found in Central Africa
    b. *Chrysomyia bezziana* (the screw-worm fly), found in Asia, Pacific, Africa and Australia
    c. *Wohlfahrtia magnifica* (the sheep maggot fly), found in Western Asia and in Russia

3. *Gasterophilidae* (horse bot or warble fly), various species, worldwide

4. *Oestridae*
    a. *Oestrus ovis* (sheep bot fly), found in Mediterranean littoral (including North Africa) and USSR
    b. *Hypoderma bovis* (cattle bot, hornet or warble fly), found in Western Asia and North Africa
    c. *Rhinoestrus purpureus* (Russian gadfly) found in South and East Europe, Western Asia and North Africa.

Ophthalmomyiasis of one kind or another has been reported in the case of each of these fly maggots on several occasions. Treatment consists of removing the maggots.

Paragonimiasis (the lung fluke)

Of several lung flukes now known to infect man, the life history of *Paragonimus westermani* is the one longest and most fully understood. Members of the cat family, pigs and dogs are the most common hosts. The adults live in the lungs and the eggs reach the outer world in the sputum, or are swallowed and passed in the stools. If they reach water, the eggs ultimately hatch motile *miracidia* which enter in turn molluscs and crustaceans. The latter (e.g. crabs, crayfish) are eaten by a definitive host or by man. From the stomach they pass to the lungs, giving rise to symptoms similar to a bronchiectasis. This parasitic disease is found in the Far East, Pacific islands, West Africa and South American, differing species being responsible.

The visual path is affected when young flukes (5 to 10 mm) invade the cerebrum or the meninges, having missed their goal (the lungs). Some become encysted; others lay eggs and others move back down the neck veins, and by the laryngopharyngeal cavity, reach the lungs or the stomach. Papilloedema and optic atrophy can result from a basal arachnoiditis originating from the encystment. Homonymous haemianopia has also been reported, as have failure of convergence and ocular palsies.

Bithionol is the drug of choice.

Pentastomiasis (tongue worm)

The larvae of *Armillifer (porocephalus) armillatus* occasionally infect humans, and ocular complications have been reported. The disease is present in Central Africa and another species, A. *moniliformis*,

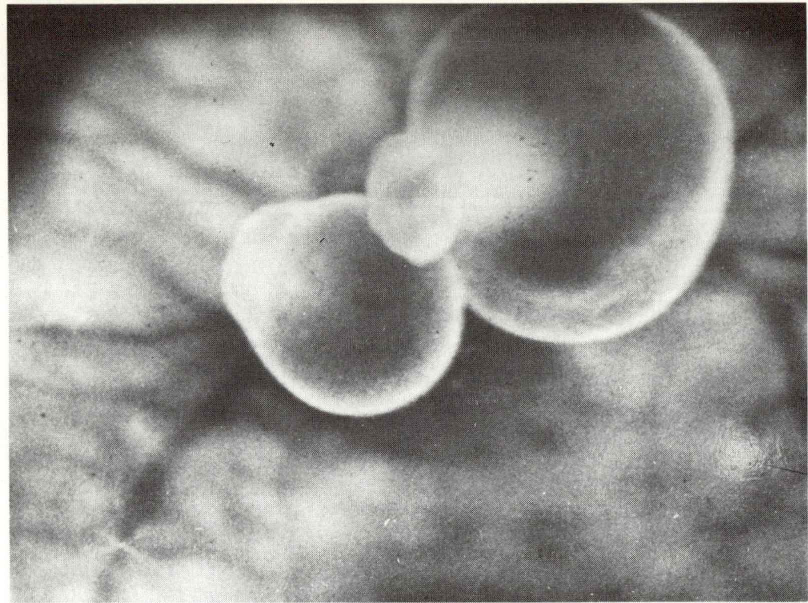

Plate 51 Cysticerci cellulosae in the fundus. Note the protruding scolex in the larger

also occurs in the Far East. The 'tongue' worms are classified somewhere between segmented worms and arthropods. The definitive hosts of the adults are snakes.

Eggs are passed by the snakes and may contaminate water; after ingestion they hatch in intermediate hosts, such as lions, baboons, giraffes and man, in whom they do not develop beyond the larval stage.

Ocular invasion is rare, but is well established as *A. armillatus* larvae (4 to 7 mm in size) have been recovered from beneath the bulbar conjunctiva and from the anterior chamber more than once. It has also been observed once in the retina, where it caused a retinal detachment, being recognised by its typical annular-ringed body, clearly visible through the retina. There is a remarkable lack of any local reaction.

Treatment consists of surgical removal.

Schistosomiasis (bilharziasis)

Schistosomiasis is the result of an infection in man by flukes of three species: *Schistosoma mansoni, Schistosoma haematobium* and *Schistosoma japonicum*. Their sizes vary from 6 to 26 mm. It is endemic on the east coast of South America, in many parts of Africa and in parts of both East and West Asia. It is estimated that 500 million people are at risk.

Eggs are excreted via the large bowel *(S. Mansoni* and *S. Japonicum)* and by the urinary bladder *(S. haematobium)*. If they contaminate fresh water in which certain snails are present, first stage mobile larvae (miracidia) will quickly develop from the eggs and penetrate the appropriate snail host. *S. mansoni* miracidia penetrate snails which are members of the genus *Biomphalaria, S. haematobium,* the snail genus *Bulinus,* and *S. japonicum,* the snail genus *Oncomelania.* Conversion of the miracidia into sporocysts occurs within the snail. Rupture of these cysts releases second stage motile larvae (cercariae) into water, where, if within a few hours they contact human skin, they can penetrate. From the dermis they migrate through the blood stream and reach the various destinations in which they develop into adults, that is in the blood vessels of the small and large intestines or bladder, depending on the species. The adults can live 10 years in man. On a global scale the incidence of schistosomiasis appears to be increasing.

During a period of systemic invasion, urticaria and oedema of the subcutaneous tissue of the lids are fairly common. Several cases of conjunctival infection have been reported from the Nile basin, a hyperendemic area for *S. haematobium,* whence most of the reports arise. Small, soft, yellowish-pink nodules appear on the conjunctiva, but have been found to contain blood-borne ova, not the larvae nor the flukes. Intraocular invasion has been reported, but surprisingly very seldom. Intracranial involvement can affect the optic nerves and visual pathway. The involvement here, too, is by reason of the eggs which are washed out of the veins in which the adults are breeding. Eggs (about 100 μm long) appear to be responsible for most of the pathological changes.

Treatment of schistosomiasis with trivalent antimony compounds is variably satisfactory, but may have to be repeated. The infection is a constant threat.

Sparganosis

Man is infected by swallowing the third stage larvae of various species of *Spirometra (diphyllobothrium) Mansoni* tapeworm. This pre-adult stage does not grow. The adult stage occurs in canines. It is found in the Far East and in Central Africa and Central America. The eggs voided into water convert to an onchosphere, are swallowed by various fresh water microcrustaceans, within which they convert to second stage larvae. The first intermediary host, the crustacean, is in turn swallowed by fish, frogs, water snakes, mammals, or by man; within all of them they alter into a third stage larva (which is known as a 'sparganum', hence the term sparganosis). A sparganum has a worm-like body and is in man from 6 to 36 cm in length, depending as always on age and sex. Man becomes infected by swallowing the parasites, either within the microcrustaceans when drinking contaminated water, or by eating the infected flesh of the intermediate host. Man, therefore, can be either a second or third intermediate host.

The fully developed spargana may enter the eye, or any body structure, directly, or can emigrate there from the alimentary tract. They cause redness, pain and oedema of the lids. Subconjunctival nodules are easily removed surgically, and confirm the diagnosis (Plate 52). Spargana also form nodules in the orbit, where they are less easily removed. As the reaction around them increases, and as the parasites increase in size within the orbit, defective closure of the lids occurs and an exposure keratitis has been recorded.

Piperazine or tetrachlorethylene therapy may be tried.

Thelaziasis (oriental eye worm)

Thelazia callipaeda is a nematode found in North West America, India and further east. It is a tiny filarial worm, 9 to 15 mm in length, and in man can be found under the conjunctiva and in the lacrimal sac. It also infects cats, dogs, deer, horses and cattle. The life cycle is unconfirmed, but the vector seems to be a fly.

The ocular symptoms may be quite painful as the worm moves around under the conjunctiva (like loa loa), causing oedema and congestion. The cornea may gradually become opaque as a result. If the worm dies, a subconjunctival parasitic tumour results. There is a single case history of a *Thelazia* worm being removed from the anterior chamber. It was the species *Th. callipaeda*. The worm should be removed surgically wherever it appears, if possible.

Diethylcarbamazine may be tried.

MYCOTIC INFECTIONS

Fungi are a large group of plantlike filamentary

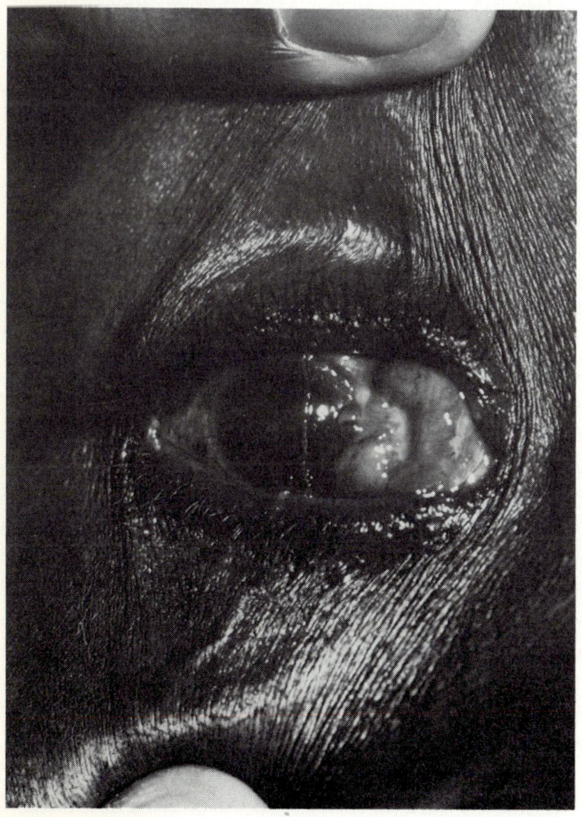

Plate 52 A subconjunctival cyst containing *Sparganum mansoni*

micro-organisms, flourishing in the soil or air, on vegetation, or even in animal products, in damp, warm and humid climates. Their filaments (hyphae) of different shapes form an interwoven mass (mycelium); this mass reproduces by spores, which either bud off from the filament or sprout from specialised hyphae. Whether the spores separate or not, they are all capable of reproducing the parent cell. If they separate they float away in the air and land on ground where there is moisture, from which they may contaminate any creature or man that may touch them. They may also be inhaled and enter the nasal sinuses or the lungs. The eye may be involved (oculomycosis) following an initial infection in its neighbourhood through a cut or abrasion of the skin, or via the orbit from the paranasal sinuses after the spores have been inhaled, or, less probably, the eye can be affected by direct transmission when the spores invade a small cut or scratch on the extraocular membranes. By reason of the fact that they are inhaled, the lungs are not infrequently simultaneously affected, giving rise to an associated systemic disorder. In addition, hypersensitivity to a fungus sometimes develops and further complicates the clinical picture.

Cases of fungal keratitis have been increasingly reported in developed countries since the introduction of antibiotics and topical steroids, especially the latter; presumably steroids suppress the immunobiological functions of the corneal cells; in this way they predispose to invasion by fungi, many of which (the air-borne) are frequently found in the conjunctival sac. Luckily only some of the many hundreds of fungi in existence appear to affect the eye of man adversely; in the absence of prolonged steroid therapy probably only a dozen are involved.

The presence of fungal infection should be suspected wherever there is a large chronic corneal ulcer, resistant to treatment, especially if the adjacent skin or the sinuses are also seen to be abnormal.

Actinomycosis

It is as well to start with actinomycosis as it is not a true fungal disease. Although it grows in colonies like fungi and forms hyphae, it tends to break up in the tissues and form free-living bacteria-like organisms. It is caused by various aerobic and anaerobic bacterial species, respectively of the genera *Nocardia* and *Streptomyces* (hence the term *Streptothricosis,* which

is now out of favour). Actinomycosis, therefore, occupies an intermediate position. The *Nocardias* are widely dispersed throughout the world and are especially common in North America, the *Streptomyces* in Africa, South America, India and the Fertile Crescent. It has also been reported recently from Vietnam.

Involvement of the lids and orbit are invariably secondary to infection of the jaw and sinuses. Primary infection conveyed through an abrasion in the skin also occurs. The cutaneous lid lesions, at first nodular, soon discharge freely. The pus contains many soft, green or yellow clumps, which are colonies or 'grains' of the fungus, the latter term describing their size. The suppurating skin lesions multiply and interconnect, and may burrow into the orbit; from here the infection may pass backwards into the posterior fossa and lead to a basal meningitis, or forwards into the lacrimal sac or gland. Concretions not infrequently are found blocking the lacrimal canaliculus, producing an intractable conjunctivitis and excessive lacrimation.

In mild ocular cases small scattered yellow nodules have been described on the palpebral conjunctiva, more usually on the bulbar conjunctiva near the limbus; both are associated with a watery, irritable eye. The conjunctival discharge is quite likely to become secondarily infected. The punctum is usually patulous and the lacrimal passage very commonly involved, because the flow of tears takes the infection into it. These changes, if untreated, can become very troublesome. A superficial punctate keratitis with pannus formation, resembling trachoma, has been described by Jones (1969).

Primary corneal ulceration, which can occur without lid involvement, due to a *Nocardia* species is rare, but has been recorded. Usually the infection does not penetrate far into the stroma and develops slowly. A corneal ulcer due to a *Streptomyces* species has been known not infrequently to follow injury. It advances steadily, has an associated hypopyon, and may perforate the eye; an exogenous endophthalmitis follows with total loss of the eye.

It is better to combine treatment with a broad spectrum antibiotic and oral dapsone 100 mg t.d.s., but this treatment has to be continued for at least 6 months. There is no certain cure. Amphotericin B locally infiltrated is disappointing. Subconjunctival injection is extremely painful, if not dangerous. Natamycin may be applied topically as a 5 per cent drop or a 1 per cent ointment every 2 hours for several days.

Aspergillosis

The entire budding body of *Aspergillus* seen under the microscope consists of a round mass of black spores on a branching stock. *A. fumigatus* and *A. niger* among many species have been isolated from ocular lesions. It is quite common in North and South America.

The mycotic agent may infect the conjunctiva, obstructing the canaliculus characteristically and leading to a dark brown discharge, but the damage done is less severe than in actinomycosis. It is known to produce corneal ulcers and very rarely has been found in the orbit, probably spreading therein from the nasal sinuses. *A. fumigatus* has been isolated from eyes with endogenous uveitis, in a few cases.

Treatment of aspergillosis consists of using nystatin eyedrops containing 10000 units per ml in normal saline, or topical nystatin eye ointment 100000 units per g, inserted every 3 or 4 hours with frequent applications of mydriatics. Subconjunctival injections of nystatin 5000 units in 0.5 ml of normal saline may be given on three separate days. Oral therapy with nystatin or Griseofulvin. has little or no effect.

Blastomycosis

In South America blastomycosis is caused by a fungus called *Paracoccidioides brasiliensis,* which grows in the tissues by budding. Primary lesions are usually in the buccal mucosa. Ulcerative granulomas extend from the nose and mouth outwards onto the skin, and inwards by metastasis to the lungs and viscera. It can lead to gross cutaneous deformities, sometimes involving the eyelids.

In North American blastomycosis, the causative organism is *Blastomyces dermatitidis,* and it also is a chronic granulomatous and suppurating disease, involving the same structures as does the South American fungus. However, it is seen as two separate types of disease: cutaneous and pulmonary (advancing to systemic).

The most common site of ocular infection by both these fungi is the eyelids, but the orbit, conjunctiva and cornea may also be involved, as may the lacrimal passages (Plate 53). There is nothing specific in the appearances.

Blastomycosis has one clinical feature not yet reported in the case of other fungi. Small nodular lesions have been found near the ciliary border of the iris and on the optic nerve. The iris nodules have been seen to break down and discharge purulent material into the anterior chamber, from which the blastomycete has been isolated.

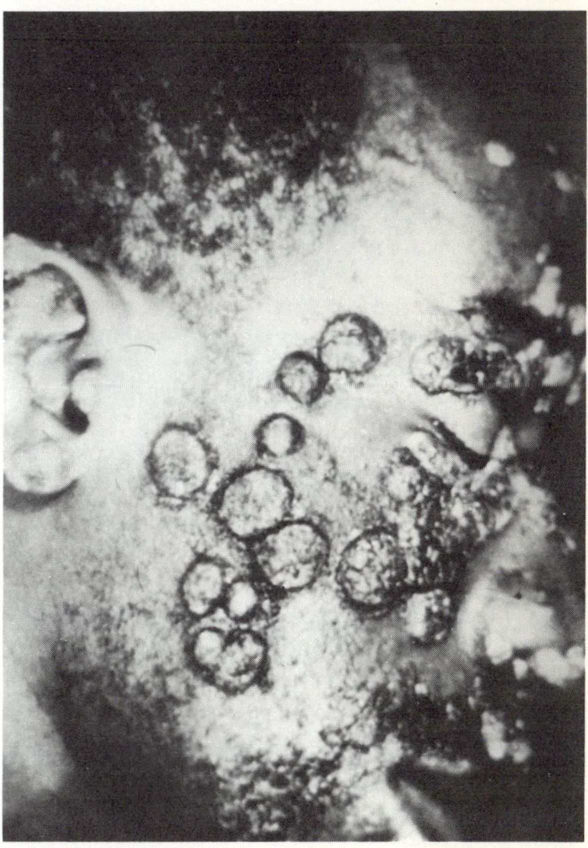

Plate 53 American blastomycosis of face and lids

Treatment of blastomycosis by long-acting sulphonamides (such as sulphormethoxine) in doses of 1 g daily have to be continued for many months, and so Amphotericin B administered in the usual way is the drug of choice: initially 0.1 mg/kg body weight is given daily over 6 hours by slow intravenous infusion, well diluted in 0.5 to 1 litre of 5 per cent dextrose in water. The dose may be increased slowly to 0.25 mg/kg, and the total dose must not be more than 2 g. Side effects include rigors and fever and impaired renal function.

Candidiosis (moniliasis, candidiasis)

The infections caused by the genus *Candida (monilia)* are characterised by their generally superficial nature and rather feeble invasive powers unless invading a wound. *C. albicans* and other species are fairly commonly present in the mouth, throat, stomach and vulva. When it attacks damaged tissues or malnourished individuals, the effect can be severe. In the malnourished the lungs may even be infected. It is a simple yeast-like fungus, which reproduces by budding. It is distributed worldwide. Of all the fungi this has been reported more frequently as an ocular pathogenic agent than any other.

C. albicans may infect the eyelids, lacrimal canals, conjunctiva and cornea, but invariably as a secondary infection, sometimes following injury, sometimes following surgery to the eye. Corneal ulceration, not infrequently in the wake of a dendritic ulcer, has been reported several times; the ulcer is described as circumscribed with a thin dry membrane on its base. A pseudo-membrane has been also described with a *Candida* conjunctivitis.

Endogenous uveitis has been only rarely described. It may be more common than believed. Following a candidaemia, an anterior uveitis occurs with extension into the anterior chamber, with hypopyon and perhaps an extension into the vitreous.

Amphotericin B is preferable to nystatin and is administered intravenously in the usual way described under Blastomycosis (above). If the patient reacts badly to this drug, 5-fluorocytosine (Flucytosine) can be used in its place. This drug is administered orally as 150 mg/kg body weight, increasing to 200 mg/kg, in four divided doses per day. One per cent fluorocytosine eye drops should be used in parallel. The total dosage by mouth should be in the neighbourhood of 220 g.

Nystatin eye ointment combined with fluorocytosine eye drops is sometimes necessary to cure a stubborn condition.

Cephalosporiosis

Various *Cephalosporium* species of this relatively benign, deep or systemic mycosis, related to penicillin, are found in man in South America, Africa and India as well as in Europe.

Cutaneous infection of the face produces deep, granulomatous areas in the dermis, from which sinuses lead to the skin's surface, and from which a mucopurulent discharge forms. In this discharge small, soft granules, somewhat similar to those in actinomycosis, are found.

Cases of infection of the lids, conjunctiva, cornea and lacrimal canals and the uvea have been reported from time to time. Always it appears to have been relatively benign compared with actinomycosis, more resembling aspergillosis; but if untreated it can lead to corneal scarring.

Treatment is with Flucytosine—or Amphotericin B should be tried.

Coccidioidosis

This infection is usually respiratory in origin, and may become disseminated throughout the body. The causative parasite is *Coccidioides immitis*. In the tissues it differs in shape from most mycoses. The basic form is a spherical cell, which never shows budding in wet preparations; it divides internally, creating a multinucleate structure, full of endospores. This grows readily in soil, the cells rupture and the endospores are disseminated in the air. It spreads by inhalation, not by touch. In general there is a benign pneumonitis in the primary infection; a more severe late hypersensitivity state develops, with a granulomatous exudate in the sputum. Frequently, especially in America, for it is found in North, Central and South America, a solitary circumscribed granuloma appears, as in tuberculosis and histoplasmosis. It may become (in the minority) a widespread, serious disease, involving the skin, with subcutaneous abscesses, going on to involve the viscera and even the meninges.

Rodents can constitute a reservoir. In addition to the Americas, a coccidioisis species is also found in the Far East.

It is somewhat rare in the external eye, but a coccidioidal granuloma of the lids has been reported several times. In such a case ocular infection involving the external eye and orbit, as in most fungal diseases of the lids, may arise. One outstanding ocular lesion, although rare, is a posterior uveitis; such a lesion, caused by coccidioidosis, has been confirmed at biopsy, non-budding cysts being present in the choroidal infiltrate. It has also been demonstrated in endophthalmitis (after enucleation). It is believed to cause a basal meningitis and produce optic atrophy when infection enters the posterior fossa from an orbital lesion.

Treatment with Amphotericin B is said to be of value.

Cryptococcosis (torulosis)

Cryptococcosis is known to be pathogenic in the Americas. It differs little in its potential spread from the mycoses previously described, causing an acute, subacute or chronic granulomatous cutaneous, pulmonary, systemic or meningeal lesion, one or all. *Cryptococcosis neoformans*, a yeast-like fungus, spreads in the blood. It is said to have various bird and mammal reservoirs. It is a sporadic infection and seems only to occur in the susceptible. It is transmitted by inhalation, reproducing by budding. It is not contagious.

It has been known to cause a typical mycotic corneal ulcer with a hypopyon. Endogenous anterior uveal infection is rare, and more likely to be seen in the terminal stage of a heavy infection; but a cryptococcal granulomatous lesion has been identified in the posterior uvea.

Involvement of the meninges and cerebrum in cryptococcosis is firmly established. The condition suggests a brain tumour, particularly because of the eye symptoms, which include papilloedema, a choked disc and optic atrophy. Involvement of the sixth nerve, leading to a convergent squint is also known to occur, as is direct invasion of the optic nerve. The organisms can be isolated in the cerebrospinal fluid.

Treatment of the systemic infection is successful with Flucytosine (see p. 106).

Fusariosis

This fungus is present in the Americas. Several authors have described mycotic corneal ulcers, with or without hypopyon, caused by *Fusarium oxysporium* and *Fusarium solani*. Corneal oedema (with a central ulcer) is so diffuse that almost the entire cornea is involved. Although it appears to be self-limiting, corneal grafting may be needed to restore sight (Polack, 1970).

Treatment with Natamycin (Pimaricin) eye drops (5 per cent suspension) is extremely well tolerated and effective.

Histoplasmosis

This widespread disease is caused by two intracellular fungi: *Histoplasma capsulatum* and the much larger *H. duboisii* (in Africa). The *Histoplasmas* grow (apparently the only fungus to do so) within the cells of the reticuloendothelial system as small, oval cells. The fungi are found in excreta in the soil, and man and some animals (baboons) and birds are infected by inhaling the spores from the earth. Direct infection does not occur. The distribution is very nearly worldwide. A smear preparation from a cutaneous lesion stained with Giemsa's or Gram's stain—it is Gram-positive—illustrates small, spheroid bodies within histiocytes (*Histoplasma cells*). They have to be differentiated from other yeast-form fungi and from Leishmanias, which they resemble.

A large number of patients have typical calcifications in the lungs and reveal allergy to tuberculin, which helps the diagnosis if such facilities are available.

The clinical course is a familiar one in mycoses. It is either a benign, subacute pulmonary infection, or localised granulomas appear on the surface of the body; cure is spontaneous. Rarely, by dissemination in the blood, a severe syndrome develops. The skin, mucous membranes, viscera and brain can become involved, and the disease may then prove fatal.

Histoplasmosis is presumed to have a partiality for the uvea. If a fungus infection elsewhere is suspected, and the posterior uvea is involved, this particular fungus must be considered. However, as *H. capsulatum* has never been isolated from the eye, it cannot be considered proven, but the clinical evidence is very suggestive, where small, discrete, multiple, peripheral areas of choroiditis, or scars, exist, with a clear vitreous, and perhaps a cystic macular lesion, adjacent to which oedema and haemorrhages are present in one or both eyes. The latter is believed to be a late specific focal reaction in tissue sensitised to the histoplasma antigen.

African histoplasmosis responds quickly to Amphotericin B and early clinical improvement, if giving empirical treatment with this drug, strengthens the diagnosis.

Mucorosis

The *Mucoraceas* are a group of fungi frequently referred to as 'bread moulds', found in the soil, manure, fruits and on starchy foods. They have a coarse, grey-white mycelium and black or brown spores. The species known as *Mucor corymbifer* has been reported in a number of instances as the cause of nasal, pulmonary and auricular mycoses, and not infrequently as the cause of an orbital cellulitis, especially in the Americas. It spreads into the orbit from the paranasal sinuses, as do so many fungi, and can advance outwards to involve the conjunctiva, lacrimal canals and sacs and the lid margins. A mucor keratitis (*M. mucedo*) has been reported *once*.

Oral potassium iodide 600 mg to 1 g in 100 ml of water t.d.s. is the treatment of choice, increasing by 300 mg/dose up to a maximum of 3 to 3.3 g/dose.

Rhinosporidiosis

The causative organism is yet another yeast-like fungus, *Rhinosporidium seeberi*, infecting the mucous membranes of the nose, mouth and eye. It causes polypus formation. It also can affect the skin, where it forms pedunculated tumours, which are soft and are formed like raspberries. It is a round organism, the cysts (sporangia) occurring in the polypoid growths between the connective tissue cells. By binary fission each sporangium becomes filled with nucleated spores, and when it bursts these spores pass via the lymphatics further afield within man's body. The disease is found in India, South America and South Africa. The exogenous method of transmission is not known, but it may be an aerosol infection.

When the face and lids are involved, rhinosporidiosis must be differentiated from yaws (framboesia), blastomycosis and leishmaniasis. Masses of pedunculated, granulomatous polyps containing the fungus produce gross, painless deformities, without—unless there is secondary infection—any discharge. The external ocular membranes and lacrimal passages are readily involved. Even the sclera has been known to be affected, with the threat of perforation of the eye.

Treatment is by excision.

Sporotrichosis

Sporothrix schenckii is the causative organism. The budding cells may be spherical or oval. It is a saprophyte causing disease in man when a cut or scratch is accidentally infected. Further invasion occurs via the lymphatics. The periorbital area is no more or no less vulnerable than elsewhere on the body's surface, and from this region the eye can be involved. Cases have been reported in tropical America and Africa.

Small, yellow, soft nodules appear on the conjunctiva in the course of the lymphatics; they eventually ulcerate and discharge pus. Perforation of the cornea or sclera with panophthalmitis occurs as a rarity. The original infective granuloma should always be sought. A few cases of endogenous granulomatous uveitis have been reported but the case needs strengthening.

Potassium iodide is specific.

Trichophytosis (ringworm)

In the tropics, ringworm occurs with various *Trichophyton* species of fungus. It may affect the skin, groin, feet, nails, scalp, ears and ocular adnexa—wherever the surfaces are damp. It has a universal distribution.

Trichophytosis quite frequently leads to a mucopurulent blepharoconjunctivitis, especially when it first has affected the moist folds of the lids. After it spreads to the lid margins an ulcerative blepharitis may continue for some time until it becomes associated with a purulent conjunctivitis. *Favus*, a severe, intractable ringworm seen in South Africa and the Far East overlaps the lids, but the conjunctiva in its case is seldom, if ever, affected.

There are many well-known treatments for cutaneous ringworm. Secondary infection of the skin may require concomitant use of an antibiotic and a steroid with a fungicide oculentum such as nystatin. As in all the mycoses, ocular treatment is generally symptomatic, for fungicidal drops are difficult to obtain and are costly.

Note on availability

The drugs mentioned above are not all commercially available, but are in the process of being produced.

SOME UNUSUAL OPHTHALMIAS

Blister beetles

The well-known drug called cantharides is prepared

from the dried bodies of *Cantharis vesicatoria* and is used on account of its blistering properties. The genus *Cantharida* contains several species with this property, known popularly as 'blister beetles', some of which are winged and some of which are not. When touched, these beetles feign death and emit a penetrating odour. The larvae of *C. vesicatoria* feed on the roots of plants.

The wings of flying blister beetles are well tolerated if they enter the eye as foreign bodies. On the other hand, if the toxic secretion of the beetle enters the eye, it produces a severe haemorrhagic belpharoconjunctivitis, which takes some days to quieten down with symptomatic treatment. The larvae have been found under the conjunctiva as a rarity.

Snake venom

In the African 'spitting' cobras, more than in any other continent, the venom contains an active haemolytic and anticoagulent factor; the main effect on the eye is local necrosis.

There are four species adapted for spitting: *Naja nigricollis nigricollis*, (in some places renamed *mossambica*), *N. nig. woodi*, and *N. nig. nigricinta*, all found in Africa; closely related to the true cobras is *Hemachatus haemachatus*, the infamous South African rinkal, which is more perfectly adapted to spitting even than the Najas. In South East Asia *N. naja* are mostly adapted for spitting though in some countries, specimens are only partly adapted. The rinkals feign death, and are not 'banded' below the throat being dark. Unlike the others their scales are 'keeled'.

The poison fangs, although comparatively short in all these species, are so constructed as to eject the venom forwards and upwards from the mouth for a distance of between 5 to 10 feet. Reid (1972) has shown that venomous snakes have two types of bite, the first being a lethal bite, inflicted to kill its prey, the second a defensive or warning bite when little or no venom is injected or expelled, the snake's object in the latter case being to escape. This probably explains why in the majority of human case histories no permanent impairment of vision is found.

N. nig. nigricollis is widespread through the Savannah regions of Africa, south of the Sahara. *N. nig. woodi* is restricted to parts of West and South West Africa. *N. nig. nigricincta* extends from South West Angola into Damaraland, South West Africa;

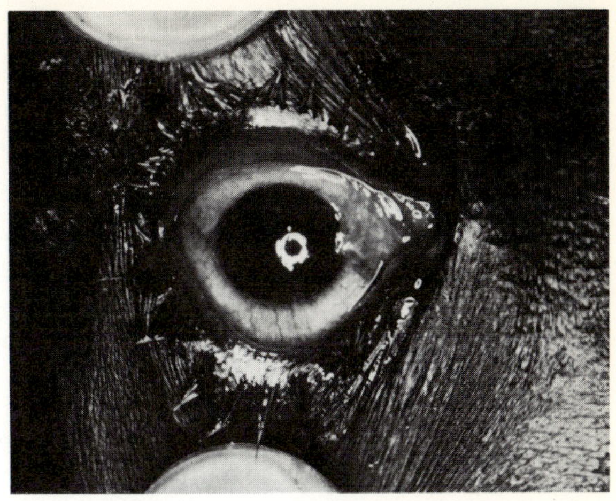

Plate 54 Snake venom ophthalmia

and the *rinkals* are restricted to South Africa and North East Zimbabwe.

Intense burning pain results when the venom strikes the external eye, and blepharospasm is severe. If the lids cannot be forced open with retractors, and the venom washed out quickly—depending, of course, on the amount present—the cornea becomes opaque and necrotic. Oedema of the lids rapidly appears and its subsidence is the first indication of recovery. Where only a small amount of venom enters the eye, sight will not be impaired, but in severe cases a white corneal scar will lead to a blind eye, very rarely bilateral. The sclera may be affected alone (Plate 54).

Wasp and bee stings

The stings of the local species of the genus *Hymenoptera* (wasps, bees and ants) in tropical countries are more severe than those in temperate climates. Wasps, being scavengers, may introduce bacteria with their stings; they have been reported to act as mechanical carriers of the eggs of *Ascaris* and *Ancylostoma*.

Most reports of bee stings to the eye have come from India, especially in the case of the giant Indian bee, *Apis dorsata*. Wasp stings in the cornea have been more frequently reported in Central America than anywhere else.

There is immediate intense ocular pain with blepharospasm; oedema and opacification of the cornea surrounding the sting develop rapidly, involving the whole corneal thickness and is frequently accompanied by an adjacent subconjunctival haemorrhage. After 24 hours a large hypopyon may arise. Raised intraocular pressure further complicates an already painful eye.

If untreated, wasp and bee sting keratitis in the absence of hypopyon and anterior uveitis, usually heals spontaneously (if slowly), leaving a leucoma. Where the sting has penetrated the cornea, on the other hand, and infection has been introduced, the eye is frequently lost.

Removal of the sting, where it has penetrated the cornea, as it is often deep, is difficult, and will require the services of an experienced ophthalmic surgeon. Despite this, an attempt should be made to remove it as soon as possible, using the slit lamp and a needle or forceps, after instilling a topical anaesthetic.

Conjunctival stings are rare.

Caterpillar hairs

Caterpillars of certain adult *Lepidoptera* possess special hairs with poison gland cells located in their bases. They are found in the tropics and subtropics. The lids may develop urticaria if these hairs become embedded. The 'saddle back' caterpillar caused numerous cases of facial and palpebral urticaria among Australian troops in Papua New Guinea in the Second World War. When such hairs accidentally enter the eye, they usually do so in numbers, giving rise to an intense reaction. They penetrate the cornea at different levels. They have been found in the posterior stroma and have been known to penetrate the cornea, being set free in the anterior chamber, or stuck in the iridocorneal angle. In some of the latter, not all, severe anterior uveitis will develop. In addition, hairs can penetrate the conjunctiva, the reaction around them producing small, vascularised nodules. If there is a solitary nodule, and this is the only abnormality found, the diagnosis is easily overlooked.

Millipede and centipede toxins

Millipedes (*Diplopoda*) are as a rule inoffensive and harmless. A large species in Fiji is known to spray a caustic fluid from special glands in the body, which causes urticaria and dermatitis upon contact with the human skin. Somewhat similar species are found in Africa. If this fluid enters the eye, a kerato-conjunctivitis develops of moderate severity. There is no authenticated record of this in point of fact from Africa, only from Fiji.

Centipedes (*Chilopoda*) are large in the tropics, especially the poisonous *Scolopendra morsitans*, which is 15 cm long. Bites are painful and by reason of the toxin injected can lead to oedema of the lids, dizziness, headache and vomiting. The poison glands are located at the base of the first pair of legs (modified to function as mouth parts) and a painful ophthalmia will ensue the moment the poison touches the external eye. *Treatment for all these conditions is symptomatic.*

7

Laboratory aids to diagnosis

This chapter has been compiled especially to help the worker, whether he is a physician, a surgeon or an ophthalmologist, who finds himself isolated in an outlying region, a doctor who wants to maintain as high a standard as he can, and who is keen to make a correct and early diagnosis. In this way sound data can be collected and a summary file compiled on the prevalence of blinding diseases in the area, more accurately than it would otherwise be. The establishment of a laboratory is further justified because it can improve the quality and efficiency of primary health care.

LABORATORY IN A SMALL UNIT

A clinician soon forgets the laboratory techniques he learned as a medical student and such techniques, the less one uses them, take on a somewhat mystical aura. Not only are the diagnostic procedures described here within the capabilities of any doctor, they are in some instances vital to diagnosis, and by enlarging the quality of his work a great stimulus.

These simple notes are only a guide and do not always complete the diagnostic process; but they offer some help to a field worker isolated by many miles from a good laboratory.

DETERMINATION OF HAEMOGLOBIN

Haemoglobin screening test

The principle is that the higher the haemoglobin level, the greater the density of a drop of blood. Copper sulphate is used because it forms a 'skin' of copper proteinate around the drop and prevents the drop from dissolving or disintegrating in the solu-tion. The concentration of the copper sulphate solutions is varied to correspond with chosen haem-oglobin levels. Although it is possible to make a series of solutions that would enable the haemoglobin level of every specimen to be estimated, it is usually sufficient to have only two solutions adjusted so that one will detect haemoglobin below 10 g/100 ml and the other below 7 g/100 ml (Standards A and B).

A stock solution of specific gravity (Sg) 1100 is made by placing 510 g of crystalline copper sulphate ($CuSO_4 5H_2O$) in a 4 litre bottle, adding 3018 ml of distilled water and shaking repeatedly to ensure complete solution. The stock solution is diluted before use: 47.2 ml made up to 100 ml with water gives an SG of 1048 (Standard A) and 41.2 ml made up to 100 ml with water gives an SG of 1042 (Stand-ard B). This should be checked with a small hydrometer if possible. The quantities apply to a temperature of 25°C and may need modifying at other temperatures. It is convenient to put 20 ml into each of 5 screw-capped universal containers and to use each bottle for no more than 20 tests.

A drop of blood taken either from a finger prick or from a venous specimen with a dropping tube is dropped vertically from a height of 1 cm into the solution. After a few seconds the blood will either rise or fall. If it rises, the haemoglobin is less than the standard.

This method is the most reliable of the simple screening tests, but depends on the concentration of plasma protein as well as the haemoglobin. If the plasma protein is less than 6.5 g/100 ml, or more than 8 g/100 ml, errors of about 5 per cent will occur.

It is sufficiently accurate for it to remain the normal method for screening blood donors for anaemia throughout the British National Blood Transfusion Service

The MRC Grey-Wedge photometer

Take up 20 μl (λ) of blood with the special pipette, making sure no bubbles are present, then add it to 4 ml of diluting fluid (0.04 per cent ammonia), first ensuring the surplus blood is wiped off the outside of the pipette. Then rinse out the pipette into the diluting fluid. Mix well. Pour into a clean cell, make sure the outside of the cell is dry, then place it in the right hand compartment of the instrument. Compare with a diluting fluid blank on the left by rotating the wheel until the two halves of the image in the eyepiece are of equal intensity. The haemoglobin is read off (rather inconveniently for modern use) in 'per cent' on the Haldane scale (100 per cent = 14.8 g/100 ml). The instrument is supplied with a standard so that a systematic error can be detected and allowed for. This method has an accuracy of ± 2 to 5 per cent, if matching is achieved by the method of 'diminishing oscillations' (described in the instrument's instruction sheet). This method uses oxyhaemoglobin which is not stable for more than 3 hours. Daylight can be used in place of batteries.

The DARE haemoglobinometer

Remove the chamber holder containing the chamber assembly from the rear of the instrument. The assembly consists of a cover glass and a grooved chamber glass. The grooved side of the chamber is against the cover, and the reverse (polished) side of the chamber points toward the nylon-tipped clamping screw. Lance the patient's finger. Allow a drop to well up. Take the chamber assembled in the holder and touch the bevelled front lips to the near side of the blood drop. Rotate the finger and chamber downward towards you. Wipe off any excess blood. Now take the assembled chamber and insert into the rear of the instrument, where you originally found this assembly. With the instrument and the scale *toward* you place an eye to the lens. Press the left thumb to switch button. Move the slide with the scale pointer with your right thumb and forefinger. Match the lower centre field to the upper centre field by the density of the colour. If the centre fields are correctly matched, then the lower left field must be denser than the upper field, and the lower right field must be less dense than the upper right field (since the upper fields are all blood sample, and the lower fields are different views along a standard wedge).

With a little experience this system assures high accuracy.

Read 'grams of haemoglobin' per 100 cc of blood from the top scale, or read 'percentage of normal haemoglobin' content from the lower 3 scales.

The chamber and the cover glass should be cleaned immediately in water, sterilised and dried.

This method has an accuracy of ± 2 g per cent Hb.

PREPARATION OF BLOOD FILMS

Thin blood films

In these films the red blood cells are discretely separated and flat, in a film one cell thick. The finger is pricked with a cutting needle, and a drop of blood placed near one end of a clean glass slide. A 'spreader slide', narrower than a normal slide, is brought *backwards* into the drop of blood at an angle of about 30°, and the spreader is then pushed forward in a steady movement, dragging a film behind it with two straight edges. The spreading of anaemic blood should be delayed a few moments, otherwise the blood film will extend right to the end of the slide. After spreading, the film is dried by waving in the air, and kept covered (or with the blood facing downwards) to prevent air-borne contamination. In a humid atmosphere the blood should be dried by warming slightly (by any convenient means), otherwise lysis of the blood may occur. When 'fixing' is required, the film is covered with methyl alcohol for at least 30 seconds.

Parasitised red blood cells tend to roll to the edges and be carried to the tail of the film, so these parts should be examined first. Haemoglobin is retained during the staining, so malaria parasites appear framed by the blood cells.

Thick blood films

In these films the red blood cells are piled thickly and irregularly. Two or three drops of blood are placed near the centre of the slide, and spread rapidly and evenly with a needle, or with the corner of another slide, into a circle about 2 cm in diameter. The final film should not be so thick that the hands of a watch cannot be seen distinctly through it. The film should be made quickly, because undue delay may lead to fibrin formation, or promote autoagglutination of red blood cells in anaemic blood. The film should be kept horizontal, and protected from dust and flies, while it dries. It should be dried as quickly as possible, preferably at 37°C. The thick blood film, being opaque to transmitted light, is made colourless by removal of the haemoglobin. Hence it is not fixed in alcohol, but is stained in an aqueous stain in which staining and lysis occur simultaneously. Alternatively, they may be stood in water for several minutes to produce haemolysis, and then dried. The outlines of the red blood cells are usually not apparent.

INTERPRETATION OF PERIPHERAL BLOOD FILMS

A good thin blood film has two straight edges and a smoothly rounded tail. With the low power objective examine the area just behind the tail and assess whether the white cells are normal, increased or decreased in number (to do this requires experience). Select an area in the centre where the red cells are seen to be evenly spaced, filling most of the field and not overlapping. Now examine this area with the oil immersion lens. Red cell appearances can be very misleading if the 'wrong' part of the film is examined.

How blood films are stained is described later. The appearances of unstained and stained films are shown in Table 7.1.

TYPICAL APPEARANCE OF SOME BLOOD FILMS

Sickle cell anaemia (SS)

White cells may be moderately increased in number,

Table 7.1 Appearances of stained and unstained blood films

Name of characteristic	Red cell appearances
Anisocytosis	The red cells vary in size more than normal
Poikilocytosis	The red cells vary in shape more than normal
Normochromia	The red cells are well-filled with haemoglobin; about 1/3 of the diameter of the cell appears pale
Hypochromia	The red cells lack haemoglobin and half or more of the cell diameters appear pale; sometimes only a narrow rim of haemoglobin is seen around the edge
Polychromasia (or diffuse basophilia)	The cells stain blueish in colour; diffusely polychromatic cells are usually reticulocytes
Punctate basophilia	Describes red cells with multiple small grey or blue dots
Spherocytosis	The cells appear smaller than normal and have no central pallor but are not crenated (wrinkled)
Macrocytosis	Most cells are larger than normal
Microcytosis	Most cells are smaller than normal. In mixed anaemias due to iron deficiency, and e.g. folate deficiency, a mixture of large and small cells may be seen—'dimorphous anaemia'
Target cells	These are cells with a rim of haemoglobin at the periphery and a lump of haemoglobin in the middle. They look therefore like targets (syn. Mexican hat cell)
Sickle cells	These are elongated, pointed and curved. They are always pathological
Pencil cells	These look similar but have square ends and are not bent and are quite often seen in iron deficiency anaemia
Kissing lip cells	These are probably sickled target cells. They have pointed ends but are not bent, and are fatter than sickled cells. They resemble pursed lips making a moue
Normoblasts	These are nucleated red cells signifying marrow over-activity. They are recognised by the haemoglobinised cytoplasm surrounding a small dark nucleus resembling that of a lymphocyte.

especially during painful crises. The red cells show marked poikilocytosis and some anisocytosis. Target cells, sickled cells, polychromatic cells and nucleated red cells may be seen. Sickled cells are often absent between haemolytic crises. The cells are *not* usually hypochromic.

Haemoglobin C disease

White cells are normal. The red cells show slight anisocytosis. There are many target cells and occasional spherocytes.

Sickle cell HbC disease

White cells usually normal. The red cells show slight anisocytosis. Target cells and occasional pseudo-sickle cells are seen: these are sickled target cells, sometimes called 'kissing lip' cells.

Iron deficiency anaemia

White cells are normal. Red cells show anisocytosis and slight piokilocytosis. Most red cells are hypochromic and microcytic. There may be a few target cells.

Thalassaemia

White cells may be slightly increased. Red cells show marked poikilocytosis, and anisocytosis (more than in simple iron deficiency). They are mainly hypochromic with (usually) many target cells. Polychromatic cells (with either diffuse or punctate basophilia) and occasional nucleated red cells are seen.

Megaloblastic anaemia

The white cells are normal or decreased in number. Many show increased lobulation of their nuclei (more than 30 per cent with five or more lobes, i.e. hypersegmentation of polymorphonuclear leucocytes). The red cells show marked poikilocytosis and moderate anisocytosis with a number of pear-shaped or 'tear-drop' cells. Most cells are macrocytic; a few polychromatic cells and nucleated cells may be seen. The red cells are *normochromic,* i.e. well-filled with haemoglobin.

In answer to the question, 'If macrocytic, is the anaemia megaloblastic?', if *not,* the cause of the anaemia is haemolysis, liver disease, aplastic anaemia, etc. If it *is* megaloblastic, the cause is folate or B12 deficiency. Failure to respond to 50 μg of vitamin B12 immediately indicates folate deficiency. The diagnostic process may have to be completed elsewhere.

DETECTION OF HAEMOGLOBIN S

The sickling test

Place a very *small* drop of blood on a clean slide, and mix it with a drop of freshly prepared 2 per cent sodium metabisulphite ($Na_2S_2O_5$) and put on a coverslip. Seal the edge of the coverslip with paraffin wax, petroleum jelly or stopcock grease. Inspect after 5 minutes, when HbSS will often have sickled. To exclude HbAS, incubate for 30 minutes at 37°C, or leave for 1 hour at ambient tropical temperature. Ignore crenated red cells. The typical sickle cell has a greater maximum diameter than a normal red cell. The speed of sickling is a very crude guide to the amount of S haemoglobin present. The tube solubility test (see below) is probably more reliable than the sickling test in detecting the sickle cell trait (heterozygote-AS).

The tube solubility test

The test is based on the principle that reduced haemoglobin S is less soluble than reduced haemoglobin A.

Place 10 mg sodium dithionite hydrosulphite ($Na_2S_2O_4$) in a small test tube (the exact amount is not critical; once the appearance of a 10 mg quantity has been appreciated, it can be imitated fairly accurately using a knife point). Add 1 ml of buffer *at room temperature* and mix. Wash in 0.02 ml (20 μl) of blood from a haemoglobin pipette (capillary or anticoagulated blood can be used). Mix by inversion, leave at room temperature and examine after 3 to 5 minutes. Reading is aided by using a background of ruled lines or fine print.

A control *normal* blood is advisable, which after 3 minutes should give a purplish solution that is transparent but *not* quite clear. A positive result for HbS is quite obvious at 3 to 5 minutes, the solution having a cloudy appearance with a flocculate appearing in a further few minutes.

It should be possible to distinguish between an SS subject and an AS after an hour or two, by which time SS will have an obvious brown precipitate while AS usually will have a marked flocculation only.

Tubes can be prepared containing the buffer and reducing reagent, which will keep in an ordinary refrigerator for about a month ready for immediate use.

Preparation of buffer (for above)

Buffer, 2.24M, pH 6.7:

Dipotassium hydrogen phosphate (K_2HPO_4)	220.3 g
Potassium dihydrogen phosphate (KH_2PO_4)	132.45 g
(NB: Weights of anhydrous salts are given here)	
Saponin	5.0 g
Distilled water to 1 litre	

STAINING BLOOD FILMS FOR PROTOZOA AND MICROFILARIAE

Several variations of the original 'polychrome' methylene blue and eosin mixture (Romanowsky stain) are available. The basic constituent of these is an eosinate of methylene blue, and in an aqueous solution this combines with the oxidation products (azures) to stain chromatin reddish-purple and cytoplasm grey-blue. The stains most commonly used in Europe are those of Leishman, Giemsa and Field; but Wright's stain (which is similar to Leishman's) is popular in America, and J.S.B. stain is much used in India and America in preference to Field's stain. Here the first three only are described for use in a small unit.

Buffered water

With Leishman's and Giemsa's stains, buffered water of pH 7.2 should be used, unless the available water is known to be neutral. To prepare buffered water, two stock solutions are needed. These are $M/15$ Na_2HPO_4 (which contains 9.5 g of disodium hydrogen phosphate in a litre) and $M/15$ KH_2PO_4 (which contains 9.07 g of potassium dihydrogen phosphate in a litre). Buffered water of pH 7.2 is prepared by mixing 72 ml of $M/15$ Na_2HPO_4, 28 ml of $M/15$ KH_2PO_4 and 900 ml of distilled water. Alternatively, a solution can be made of 0.7 g of KH_2PO_4 and 1.0 g of Na_2HPO_4 in 1 litre of distilled water.

The solutions should be stored in hard glass (Pyrex) stoppered bottles. It is possible to obtain buffer tablets to give the required pH, but these are relatively expensive.

Leishman's stain (for protozoa in thin blood films)

This stain consists of the combined precipitate of polychrome methylene blue and eosin, dried and then dissolved in methyl alcohol. The stain is bought as a powder. 0.15 g of stain is triturated in 100 ml of methyl alcohol at 37°C. It is ready for use after 24 hours, after filtering. The stock solution should be kept in a well-stoppered glass bottle in subdued light, or the stain will rapidly deteriorate.

Leishman's stain is used for *thin blood films only*. Two pipettes are required, one for the alcoholic stain and one for the buffered water. Standardisation of results is obtained by having the pipettes graduated to deliver 0.5 ml and 1.5 ml. 0.5 ml of stain is placed on the horizontal slide, with the blood film upwards. The stain will fix the blood in 30 seconds. Now 0.5 ml of buffered water (pH 7.2) is added, and the mixture left for 8 to 10 minutes for staining malaria, spirochaetes or trypanosomes, or 15 minutes for staining leishmanias in tissue smears. The stain is then flooded off with running water for a few seconds only, and the slide is placed at an angle to dry. If prolonged washing is given, the water-soluble methylene blue will be removed and the cytoplasm of the parasites left unstained.

Giemsa's stain I (for protozoa in thin blood films)

This stain is usually bought as a solution, but it can be prepared by mixing 3.8 g of Giemsa powder with 250 ml of methyl alcohol and 250 ml of glycerine. The powder is placed in a mortar and ground thoroughly, and the glycerine is added to the mortar a little at a time, grinding and mixing taking place with each addition. About half the methyl alcohol is then added, and also ground and mixed; and the contents of the mortar are then poured into a glass-stoppered Pyrex bottle. The remainder of the methyl alcohol is then poured into the mortar, and mixed and ground with the residue of the stain. The whole contents of the mortar are then poured into the bottle, and the mixture is incubated for 24 hours at 37°C, giving the bottle an occasional shake. The stain is filtered into dropping bottles before use.

The stain is used after dilution with buffered water, and therefore preliminary fixation of *thin blood films* is necessary. *Thin films should be fixed in methyl alcohol for at least 30 seconds and then stained in a 10 per cent solution of Giemsa's stain in buffered water.* Single films are stained face downwards on a curved staining plate, large numbers of films in a staining trough, for 20 to 30 minutes. The stain is then washed off, and the slides are dried by placing them at an angle. They must not be blotted.

Giemsa's stain II (for protozoa and mf. in thick films)

The *thick* film is dried at room temperature or at 37°C, *not* fixed, and then stained for 1 hour in a 3 per cent solution of Giemsa's stain in buffered water (pH 7.2). The film is stained and lysed simultaneously. The film is then washed *carefully* but *rapidly* at an angle in air. This staining method is useful where both *W. bancrofti* and *B. malayi* are endemic, because differential staining of these species occurs. The sheath of *Mf. Bancrofti* stains blue, of *Mf. Malayi pink*. The stained film can also be used for diagnosis of malaria, using the X100 objective. The *Mf. loa* sheath takes up hardly any stain at all, and looks clear.

Mayer's acid haemalum stain (for mf. in skin snips and thick blood films)

This stain is prepared by first dissolving 2 g of haematoxylin crystals in 10 ml of alcohol. Fifty g of potassium aluminium sulphate is then dissolved in hot water and to this solution is added the haematoxylin solution and also 0.2 g of sodium iodate. The solution is then made up to 1 litre with distilled water. When the solution has cooled, add a crystal of thymol and 20 ml of glacial acetic acid. The stain can be obtained ready made up and keeps quite well in the field for a month.

A thick blood film, dehaemoglobinised in water, dried and fixed in methyl alcohol for 1 minute, and a skin snip, dried and fixed in methyl alcohol, are stained with Mayer's for 3 to 10 minutes. The stain is heated until it steams before being washed off by plunging into water, although mf. nuclei can be seen without heating, if less clearly. Prolonged washing 'blues' the nuclei of mf. A spirit burner is a good source of heat. (This stain can also be used directly on urinary sediment.

Preservation of stained blood films

Any immersion oil on the film should be carefully removed with xylol. When the slide is dry, apply a drop of neutral mounting medium and cover with a No. 1 coverslip. This will protect the film from dust and scratches. Deterioration may occur quickly in the tropics, and films should not be left exposed to sunlight.

STAINING FOR BACTERIA AND FUNGI

Gram's stain (for bacteria and fungi)

Nearly all bacteria will take up methyl violet, and most fungi. This stain can be 'mordanted' (made fast) with iodine only in certain groups of bacteria (Gram-positive), but not in others (Gram-negative) (Table 7.2). The iodine must be dark.

Table 7.2 Gram-positive and -negative organisms

Gram-positive		*Gram-negative*
Cocci	Staphylococcus	Neisseria meningitidis
	Streptococcus	Gonococcus
	Pneumococcus	(Catarrhalis spp. are
		commensals)
Bacilli	Anthrax	Pseudomonas pyocyanea
	Clostridium (the	Haemophilus influenzae
	anaerobic bacilli	Salmonella
	including gas gangrene)	Bacterioides
	Diphtheroids	Escherichia coli
	Acid-fast group	Proteus vulgaris
	Many fungi	

Acetone treatment of these stained films will than remove methyl violet from Gram-negative bacteria but not from Gram-positive, which are mordanted and stay purple. A final counterstain of safranin will stain the decolourised Gram-negative bacteria *red*. The Gram-positive bacteria remain *purple*.

Method

1. Make a thin bacterial film and fix
2. Place cooled slide on sink rack. Cover with methyl violet 1 min
3. Wash off methyl violet with water. Drain off residual water. Cover film with iodine soln 1 min
4. Wash off iodine with water. Tip off completely
5. Holding the slide, quickly pour acetone across the film and immediately move the slide into running tap water. Rinse thoroughly
6. Tip off water. Cover film with safranin ½ min
7. Wash off safranin with water. Drain slide quickly. Gently blot dry—avoid rubbing film but clean back of slide
8. Examine dry stained film by oil immersion microscopy.

Ziehl-Neelsen's stain (for mycobacteria)

Mycobacteria have a thick waxy coat which is not penetrated by ordinary stains. Hot, strong carbol fuchsin will penetrate and stain mycobacteria red. The test is made specific for mycobacteria as follows:

1. *All* bacteria will take up the hot strong stain, but
2. Only mycobacteria (because of the waxy coat) resist decolourisation, because while all mycobacteria are *acid*-fast, some of the relatively unimportant commensal mycobacteria are decolourised by *alcohol*, whereas *Myco. tuberculosis* is not, i.e. *Myco. tuberculosis* is *acid-alcohol* fast
3. A blue counterstain then shows:
      non-mycobacteria = non acid-fast = blue
      mycobacteria   = acid-fast   = red

Method

1. Prepare a thin film and fix thoroughly by heat
2. Flood slide with strong carbol fuchsin
3. Heat gently till the stain begins to steam. *Do not boil.*
   Add more stain as necessary to prevent drying. Keep steaming for 5 minutes
4. Wash well with water
5. Treat with 25 per cent sulphuric acid for a total of 10 minutes, changing the acid 2 or 3 times during this period

6. Wash well with water. The film should now appear a *very* faint pink
7. Treat with 95 per cent alcohol for 2 minutes. Wash off
8. Treat with methylene blue counterstain for 30 seconds. *Wash well* with water. Blot and dry.

Modifications for M. leprae. Stain for 10 minutes with strong carbol fuchsin. For decolourising, use a solution of 1 per cent sulphuric acid in alcohol. Strong acid as used for *Myco. tuberculosis* will decolourise *M. leprae* completely.

CEREBROSPINAL FLUID

Technique of lumbar puncture

Lumbar puncture is carried out using one of several lumbar puncture needles, such as the Harris. The patient lies in the fetal position at the edge of the bed and a small bleb (0.15 ml approx) produced by injecting a local anaesthetic just beneath the skin; trauma will result if a deeper injection is given. The needle is inserted between the third and fourth lumbar vertebrae. A line joining the highest points of the iliac crests usually passes between the third and fourth lumbar spinous processes. The needle is passed forwards and slightly upwards in mid-plane. At a depth of 4 to 5 cm the needle point has to pass through the ligamentum flavum (which requires a little pressure), and after penetrating a further 0.50 cm, should enter the subarachnoid space. The stylet is now withdrawn and three samples of 3 ml are obtained in separate glass bottles from the butt end of the needle. The patient is then left lying face down for an hour to prevent headache.

The appearance of the c.s.f. (clear, turbid) is helpful. Microscopic examination, unstained or stained, with Gram's, will demonstrate the presence or absence of infection and the type.

Significance of appearance

Yellowish discolouration with blood may be present in the c.s.f. either due to the needle (in which case the second and third 3 ml specimen should have progressively less discolouration), or due to a pre-existing subarachnoid haemorrhage (in which all three will be coloured equally). If normal, c.s.f. resembles water. Turbidity is usually due to an excess of polymorph cells and protein. If yellowish or turbid, the c.s.f. should be spun in a hand centrifuge and the sediment examined for red or white cells. In certain virus infections (e.g. herpes, Coxackie, etc.) the c.s.f. appears clear.

White cell count

Place two drops of well-mixed c.s.f. into a small test tube. Fill one side of a double counting chamber (improved Neubauer) with the c.s.f. remaining in the Pasteur pipette used (undiluted c.s.f.). Take some white blood cell diluting fluid into a Pasteur pipette. Add two drops to the two drops of c.s.f. in the small test tube. Mix well by drawing in and out of the pipette. Any red cells present will be lysed and the white cells stained a pale blue.

Fill the second half of the counting chamber with the c.s.f white cell fluid mixture (diluted c.s.f.).

Results as cells/mm³

1. Undiluted c.s.f:

many cells –   count the cells in 16 small squares and multiply the answer by 10.

few cells –   count the cells in all parts of the chamber and in one extra block of 16 small squares: this will be 1mm³ and there is no need to do any multiplying.

2. Diluted c.s.f:

many cells –   count as for undiluted c.s.f. above, but multiply the answer by 20 instead of 10.

few cells –   count as for undiluted c.s.f. but multiply answer by two.

Normally there are less than 4 w.b.c./mm²

Sugar

'Dip-strip' testing for sugar, protein and blood is a rough but simple technique (see p. 119). Protein is high and sugar absent in cerebrospinal meningitis.

Pandy's qualitative test for c.s.f. protein

Mix the c.s.f. well with a glass rod. Add two drops of c.s.f. to a Kahn tube half-filled with Pandy's reagent. Normal c.s.f. produces no turbidity. If there is an abnormal amount of protein in the c.s.f., a 'smoky trail' is visible and the Pandy's reagent will go turbid on mixing. Record the turbidity with the plus notation:

No turbidity—negative result   –ve
Very slight turbidity (just visible) +
Obvious turbidity   ++
Complete flocculation   +++

Pandy's test will not show a positive result until the c.s.f. protein exceeds 100 mg/100 ml, above which inflammatory disease of the meninges is almost certain, although intracranial tumours, an acoustic neuroma and a cerebral infarction can cause a rise in protein content.

Further protein tests

Gallenkamp proteinometer

Three ml of 3 per cent sulphosalicylic acid is placed in a glass tube and 1 ml of c.s.f. added. Leave for 3 minutes and then the turbidity is compared with a set of standards.

Globulin

Two to 3 ml of saturated ammonium sulphate (aqueous solution) is placed in a test tube and c.s.f. slowly added. A white precipitate at the interface is positive for the presence of globulin.

URINE ANALYSIS

Reagent tests

Protein

Place 5 ml of urine in a 6 + ½ in test tube. Boil the upper third of the urine. Add 6 to 8 drops of 33 per cent acetic acid quickly. Turbidity in the upper layer indicates the presence of protein.

Sugar

To 0.5 ml of urine in a test tube, add 5 ml of Benedict's qualitative reagent. Place in a boiling water bath for 5 minutes, or boil vigorously over a flame for 1 minute, then allow to cool.

Observe any colour change:

green —0.25
yellow —0.50
orange—1.00 } per cent reducing substance
brick —2.00
red

Note: 1. This test detects reducing substances and is not specific for glucose.
2. A white or greyish precipitate of phosphate may sometimes appear and simulate a feeble reaction.
3. If this test is positive but the glucose 'dip-strip' test is negative, suspect either galactosuria or that the 'dip-strip' test has deteriorated.

'Dip-strip' tests

The test selected and recommended is the BM-Test (Boehringer Mannheim). These are made up in packs of 50 strips, which in a cool, dark place should last 18 months.

The BM-Test 5 strip for nitrite, glucose, protein, urobilinogen and blood is dipped in fresh urine up to each mark for no longer than one second. Wipe off excess urine on the rim of the vessel. After 30 to 60 seconds the test patches are compared with the colour scale on the container. Changes of colour appearing only along the edges of each test patch, or after more than 2 minutes, are of no significance. There are other, more complex (and more expensive) strips.

Urinary sediment

A hand centrifuge (with two tubes each ¾ full) is spun for 2 to 3 minutes. The supernatent is decanted. A few drops of methanol are allowed to fall on the sediment in the tube, which is then inverted. The contents are then tipped onto a glass slide, allowed to dry well in the air and covered for study later. Alternatively, some sediment can be placed on a glass slide with a pipette and fixed by heat (or methyl alcohol) before being stained by Gram's or Mayer's acid Haemalum.

In women, *trichomanas* is a common urinary contaminant, as is *enterobius*. Mites may be also accidental contaminants.

Mf. volvulus can be found in the centrifuged sediment, as can the eggs of *Schistosoma haematobium* (with a terminal spine) and, rarely, those of *S. mansoni* (with a lateral spine). These parasites plus cells, crystals and casts can be seen by direct microscopy.

SKIN

Skin biopsies (for mf. volvulus)

A fine hypodermic needle is passed under the dermis for 1 cm and the end (held between the fingers) raised so the skin is stretched. A razor blade shaves off a small piece of skin (which is weighed in comparative studies). Placed on a glass slide in a drop of distilled water it is teased out and a cover slip is placed over the skin biopsy. It is put aside for up to ½ hour, by which time all mf. should have emerged. They are then counted under a microscope. If necessary they may be stained later in the laboratory, identified and then counted in case blood-borne mf. have contaminated the specimen. Mayer's stain is the author's choice.

Skin scarifications (for skin and blood mf.)

Scarifications for all filarial mf. may be carried out with any sharp instrument, e.g. a vaccination lancet, or with a hypo needle. One cm^2 of skin is scarified and the scrapings placed on a glass slide for examination and counting later after staining. The usual sites are in the scapular and trochanteric regions. Giemsa's stain gives good results.

FUNGAL EXAMINATION

A scraping of the suspect tissue is placed on a slide. Fifteen per cent potassium hydroxide is dropped on the material and the tissue gently teased. The characteristic hyphae and spores should be readily visible, if present, by direct microscopy.

THE HEAF TEST

The Heaf gun is an instrument with a spring which

suddenly forces 6 sharp needles into the skin when its trigger mechanism is activated. The test is performed on the volar surface of either forearm. One drop of undiluted OT or PPD in a strength of 2 mg/ml is spread on a clean area of skin and the Heaf gun needles triggered through the drop while it is still wet. The depth of protrusion of the needles beyond the guard plate on the gun can be adjusted to 1 mm for small children and to 2 mm for older subjects. The result is inspected after 2 to 7 days and recorded as described in the final Table.

Before applying the gun to each patient, the instrument is sterilised by dipping the needles in alcohol and igniting the alcohol. If this is not done there is a theoretical danger of transmitting infectious hepatitis or syphilis. A false positive result can be caused by using the instrument when it is still hot enough to burn the skin or by carbon deposits on the needles.

A grade 3 or 4 response (see below) is a definite positive. A Heaf grade 2 is probably positive and a grade 1 is probably negative.

STOOLS

Stool examination is not stressed for, if negative, several specimens will have to be examined and this is time consuming and frequently unrewarding to the lone worker. Moreover, it requires many years of experience to sort out the mixture of parasites and saprophytes found in faeces. Direct saline and iodine preparations can be utilised if the microscopist has experience and knowledge of the various protozoa and ova likely to be present.

ERYTHOCYTE SEDIMENTATION RATE (ESR)

The well-known Westergren method is easy to carry out, but the author has found little use for this test in tropical ophthalmology; temperatures above 20°C affect the result variously, as do pregnancy, menstruation and some anaemias. Reduction in the ESR occurs in the sickle cell diseases and haemolytic anaemias.

Interpretation of Heaf Reactions

Grade 0	4 palpable papules	Negative
Grade 1	4 to 6 palpable papules	Possibly cross-sensitisation
Grade 2	A discrete circle of induration	Probably positive
Grade 3	A palpable plaque with the centre of the circle filled	Definitely positive
Grade 4	A palpable plaque with vescicles (surrounding erythema is ignored)	

References

Anderson DR, Braverman S 1976 Re-evaluation of the optic disk vasculature. American Journal of Opthalmology 82: 165–174

Arita J 1979 Virological evidence for the success of the smallpox eradication programme. Nature 279: 293–298

Atias A, Schilling E, Naquira N, Valenzuele R 1963 A fatal congenital case of Chaga's disease. Bolivia–Chile Parasitology 18: 14–16

Bietti GB, Oomen HAPC, Rodger FC, Winkler PG 1972 Prevention of blindness. Technical Report Series, WHO Publications, Geneva

Bird AC, Anderson J, Fuglsang H 1976 Morphology of posterior segment lesions of the eye in patients with onchocerciasis. British Journal of Ophthalmology 60: 2–20

Blumenthal CJ 1950 Malnutritional keratoconjunctivitis of S. African Bantu. South African Medical Journal 24: 191–198

Brewerton DA 1977 In: Perkins ES, Hill DW (eds) Scientific foundations of opthalmology, Heinemann Medical, London pp 100–102

Brontë-Stewart J, Pettigrew AR, Foulds WS 1976 Toxic optic neuropathy and its experimental production. Transactions of the ophthalmology society UK 96: 355–358

Browne SG 1979 Personal communication

Buck AA (ed) 1974 Onchocerciasis. WHO Publication, Geneva

Chatterjee S, Quarcoopome CO, Apenteng A 1970 Unusual type of epidemiological conjunctivitis in Ghana. British Journal of Ophthalmology 54: 628–630

Crewe W, Wéry M 1977 In: Rodger FC (ed) Onchocerciasis in Zaire. Pergamon Press, Oxford. pp 80–81

Croizier RC 1968 Traditional Medicine in Modern China. Harvard University Press, Cambridge, USA

Dean Hart JC, Raistrick ER 1977 Adult toxocariasis. Transactions of the Ophthalmology Society UK 97: 164–167

Douglas GR, Drance SM, Schulzer M 1974 The visual field and nerve head following acute angle closure glaucoma. Canadian Journal of Ophthalmology 9: 404–407

Duke-Elder S, Perkins ES 1966 System of Ophthalmology, vol IX. Henry Kimpton, London p 246

Florman AL, Agatston HJ 1962 Keratoconjunctivitis as a diagnostic aid in measles. Journal of the American Medical Association 179: 568–570

Foerster HW 1959 Granulomatous uveitis in man and experimental animals. Survey of Ophthalmology (USA) 4: 283–326

Galbraith JEK 1979 Basic eye surgery. Churchill Livingstone, Edinburgh

Hakim SAE 1954 Argemone oil, sanguinarine and epidemic dropsy glaucoma. British Journal of Ophthalmology 38: 193–216

Houwer AWM 1946 Amblyopia cum polyneuropathia caused by starvation. Ophthalmologica (Basel) 112: 177–192

International Classification of Diseases: Blindness 1979 WHO Geneva

IVACG Report 1976 Guidelines for the Eradication of Vitamin A Deficiency and Xerophthalmia: a report of the International Vitamin A consultative Group

Jelliffe D 1961 see Nicholls (1938)

Jones BR 1969 Antifungal drugs for oculomycosis. Transactions of the Ophthalmology Society UK 89: 819–835

Jones BR 1977 In: Perkins ES, Hill DW (ed) Scientific Foundations of Ophthalmology Heinemann Medical, pp 149–159

Jones BR, Falcon MG, Williams HP, Coster DJ 1977 Objectives in Therapy of herpetic eye diseases. Transaction of the Ophthalmology Society UK 97: 305–313

Kende AD 1970 In: Polack FM (ed) Corneal and External Diseases of the Eye. Thomas, Springfield, Ill. pp 71–85

King JH, Passmore JW 1955 Nutritional amblyopia: a study of American prisoners of war in Korea. American Journal of Ophthalmology 39: 173–186

Leader Stirling, Opening Address, Seminar on Malaria Control, Dar es Salaam, 1979

MacCallan AF 1931 Epidemiology of trachoma. British Journal of Ophthalmology 15: 369–411

Michaelson IC 1968 Medical help to developing countries. World Hospitals 4: 59–62

Miller SJH 1977 In: Perkins ES, Hill DW (eds) Scientific foundations of opthalmology. Heinemann Medical, London, pp. 72–75

Mojon M 1977 In: Rodger FC (ed) Onchocerciasis in Zaire. Pergamon Press, Oxford. pp 85–103

Nicholls 1938 Tropical Nutrition and Dietetics, Sinclair HM, Jelliffe DB (rev in 1961) Baillière, Tindall & Cox, 4th edn.

Nizetic B 1975 Public health ophthalmology. In: Hobson W (ed) Theory and Practice of Public Health. Oxford University Press, London

Pirie NW 1978 Leaf Protein and other Aspects of Fodder Fractionation. Cambridge University Press, London

Polack FM 1970 In: Corneal and External Diseases of the Eye, 1st International American Symposium. Thomas, Springfield, Ill. pp 53–66

Reid HA 1972 Snake bite. Tropical Doctor 2: 155–163

Rodger FC 1952 Nutritional amblyopia: a report on Japanese prisoners of war. Archives of Ophthalmology (Chicago) 47: 570–583

Rodger FC 1959 Blindness in West Africa. Lewis, London. Ch 3, 6

Rodger FC 1963 A reappraisal of the ocular lesion known as Bitot's spot. British Journal of Nutrition 17: 475–485

Rodger FC 1973 The effect of heavy parasite loads (of 0. volvulus) on human optic nerve. Helminthologia (Praha) 14: 39–49

Rodger FC 1973 Bietti's corneal degeneration in the Dahlak Islands. British Journal of Opthalmology 57: 657–664

Rodger FC 1976 A miniature clinical and field dark adaptometer with a tritium light source. American Journal of Ophthalmology 82: 313-315

Rodger FC, Farooqi HU 1959 Lesions of the lid margins caused by ectoparasites in India. British Journal of Ophthalmology 43: 676–680

Rodger FC, Sinclair HM 1969 Metabolic and nutritional eye disease. Thomas, Springfield, Ill. Chap. 5

Rodger FC, Cuthill JA, Fydelor PJ, Lenham AP 1974 UVR as a possible cause of corneal degenerative changes under certain physiographic conditions. Acta Ophthalmologica 52: 777–785

Rodger FC, Maertens K 1977 In: Rodger FC (ed) Onchocerciasis in Zaire. Pergamon Press, Oxford, pp. 105–139

Sinclair HM 1961 see Nicholls (1938)

Slansky HH 1970 In: Polack FM (ed) Corneal and external diseases of the eye. Thomas, Springfield, Ill. pp 147–153

Tarizzo ML 1973 Field Methods for the Control of Trachoma. WHO Publications, Geneva p 9

Ticho U, Ben-Sira I 1970 Nonpigmented tumors of the conjunctiva and pingueculas among Africans. American Journal of Ophthalmology 70: 757–763

Wadsworth GR 1977 In: Rodger FC (ed) Onchocerciasis in Zaire. Pergamon Press, Oxford. Ch 3

Wilcocks C, Manson-Bahr PEC 1972 Manson's Tropical Diseases 17th edn. pp 247, 559–565

Wilder HC 1951 Nematode endophthalmitis. Transactions of the Academy of Ophthalmology and Otolaryngology 55: 99–109

Wilson WA, Graham RVH 1979 Rheumatic disease in Jamaica. Annals of Rheumatic Diseases 38: 320–325

Woods AC 1961 Endogenous inflammation of the Uveal Tract. Williams & Wilkins Co, Baltimore

Index

Names and initials in italics refer to authors mentioned in the text